CW00855468

Around the British Isles in 80 Races

by

Dave King

AuthorHouse™ UK Ltd.
500 Avebury Boulevard
Central Milton Keynes, MK9 2BE
www.authorhouse.co.uk
Phone: 08001974150

First published by AuthorHouse 10/30/2008

ISBN: 978-1-4343-6555-2 (sc)

Printed in the United States of America
Bloomington, Indiana

This book is printed on acid-free paper.

To

Micah, Leo and Ross

Live your dreams and let no-one take them away from you - you are the inspiration to my perspiration!

WHERE IT ALL HAPPENED

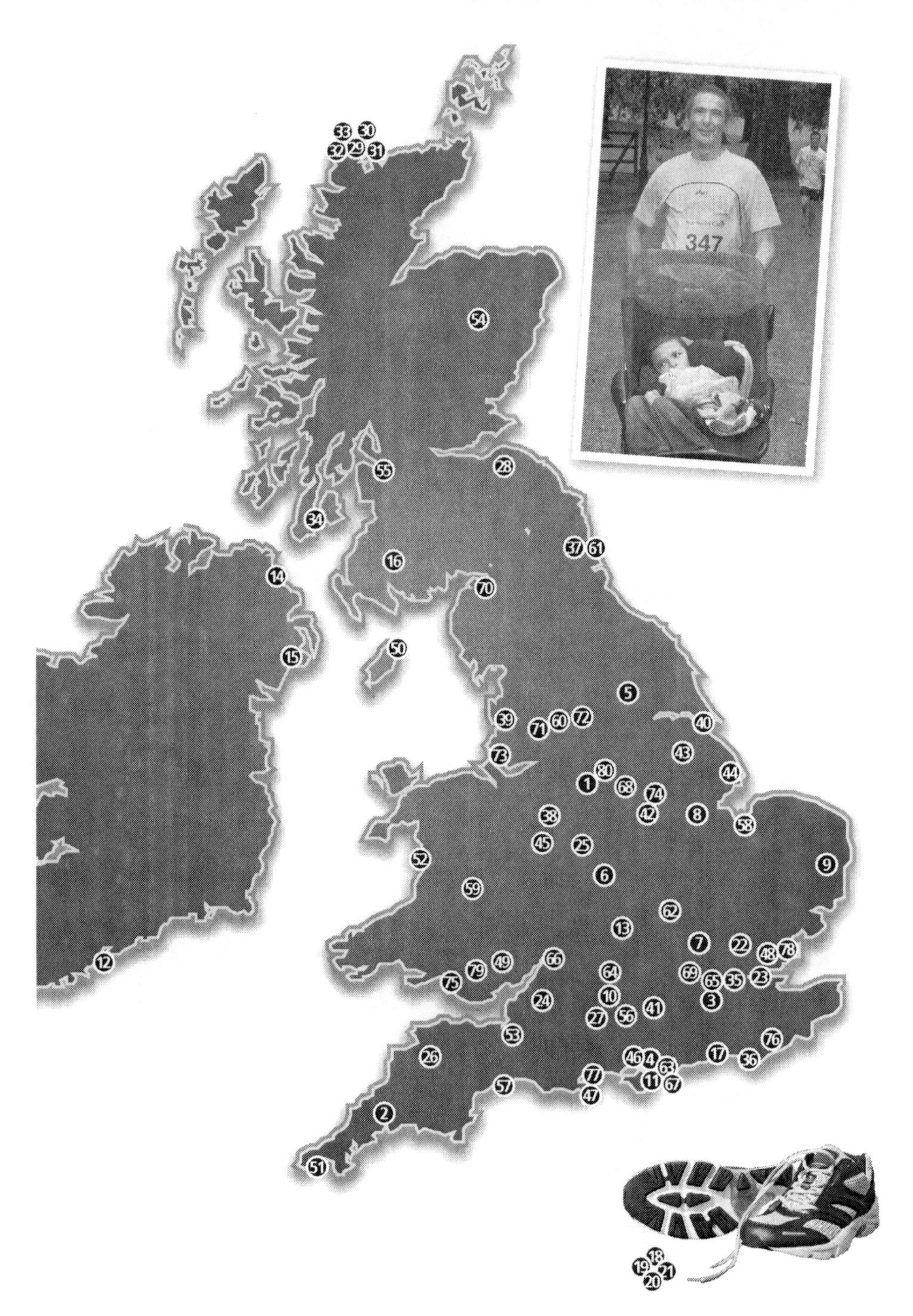

WHERE IT ALL HAPPENED

Around the British Isles in 80 races

1. December 31st, 2006: **Bryan Clifton Memorial Midnight Run** @ Milford Derbyshire. (2km)

JANUARY 2007

2. January 1st, 2007: **Brown Willy 6** @ Bodmin Moor, Cornwall. (6.8 miles)
3. January 7th: **Tadworth 10** @ Epsom Downs, Surrey. (10 miles)
4. January 14th: **Stubbington Green 10km** @ Stubbington, Hampshire. (10km)
5. January 21st: **Brass Monkey Half Marathon** @ York, North Yorkshire. (13.1 miles)
6. January 28th: **Not The Roman IX** @ Stratford-upon-Avon, Warwickshire. (7.4 miles)

FEBRUARY

7. February 4th: **Asics Watford Half Marathon** @ Watford, Hertfordshire. (10 miles)
8. February 11th: **Stamford Striders' St Valentine 30km** @ Stamford, Lincolnshire. (30km)
9. February 18th: **Great East Run** @ Bungay, Suffolk. (20km)
10. February 25th: **The Terminator** @ Pewsey, Wiltshire. (11.5 miles)

MARCH

11. March 1st: **Vectis Lunatics' Full Moon Run** @ Ryde, Isle of Wight. (3.5 miles)
12. March 4th: **Ballycotton 10** @ Ballycotton, County Cork, Republic of Ireland. (10 miles)
13. March 11th: **Banbury 15** @ Banbury, Oxfordshire. (15 miles)
14. March 17th: **Glenariff Mountain Race** @ Waterfoot, County Antrim, Northern Ireland (6 miles)
15. March 18th: **Jimmy's 10** @ Downpatrick, County Down, Northern Ireland. (10km)
16. March 24th: **Asics Coniston 14** @ Coniston, Cumbria (14 miles)

APRIL

17. April 1st: **Worthing 20** @ Worthing, West Sussex. (20 miles)
18. April 6th: **Guernsey Easter 10km road race** @ Port Soif, Guernsey. (10km)
19. April 7th: **Guernsey Easter cross country** @ L'Ancresse, Guernsey (4 miles)
20. April 8th: **Guernsey Easter 4x2 mile relay** @ L'Ancresse, Guernsey. (2 miles)
21. April 9th: **Guernsey Easter Half Marathon** @ St Peter Port, Guernsey. (13.1 miles)
22. April 15th: **Flitwick 10km** @ Flitwick, Bedfordshire (10km)
23. April 22nd: **Flora London Marathon.** (26.2 miles)
24. April 29th: **Horton Bull Run** @ Chipping Sodbury, Gloucestershire. (4 miles)

MAY

25. May 2nd: **Dudley Kingswinford 10km** @ Dudley, West Midlands. (10km)
26. May 4th: **Round the Tree 3** @ Torrington, Devon (3 miles)
27. May 6th: **Neolithic Cani-X** @ Stonehenge, Wiltshire. (4 miles)
28. May 12th: **Penicuik 10km** @ Penicuik, Midlothian. (10km)
May 14th – May 19th: **Cape Wrath Challenge** @ Durness, Scotland.
29. May 14th: **Half Marathon: Loch Eriboll to Durness**, Sutherland. (13.1 miles)
30. May 15th: **Sangomore Hill Run** @ Durness, Sutherland. (5 miles)
31. May 16th: **Durness Run** @ Durness, Sutherland. (8.4 miles).
32. May 17th: **Target Zero Beach Run** @ Durness, Sutherland. (3 miles)
33. May 19th: **Marathon Relay** @ Durness, Sutherland. (13.1 miles)
34. May 27th: **Mull of Kintyre Half Marathon** @ Campbeltown, Mull of Kintyre. (13.1 miles).
35. May 28th: **Beat the Baton** @ Battersea Park, London. (5km).

JUNE

36. June 2nd: **South Downs Way Relay** – Beachy Head, East Sussex to Chilcomb, Hampshire. (16.5 miles over 3 legs)
37. June 9th: **Blaydon Races** @ Blaydon, Tyneside. (5.7 miles)
38. June 10th: **Asics Potters Arf** @ Stoke-on-Trent, Staffordshire. (13.1 miles)
39. June 17th: **Freckleton Half** @ Freckleton, Lancashire. (13.1 miles)
40. June 24th: **Humber Bridge Half Marathon** @ Hull, Humberside. (13.1 miles)
41. June 27th: **Army Orienteering Association race** @ Longmoor Camp, Hampshire. (4.5 miles)

JULY

42. July 1st: **Prestwood Hall 10k** @ Prestwood, Leicestershire (10km).
43. July 7th: **Tickhill Gala Run** @ Tickhill, South Yorkshire. (3.5 miles)
44. July 8th: **Spilsby Show 6** @ Spilsby, Lincolnshire. (6 miles)
45. July 15th: **Wenlock Olympian Games** @ Much Wenlock, Shropshire. (7 miles)
46. July 21st: **Mug's Game 5** @ Itchen Valley Country Park, Eastleigh, Hampshire. (4.5 miles)
47. July 28th: **Swanage Half Marathon** @ Swanage, Dorset. (13.1 miles)

AUGUST

48. August 5th: **Harlow 10** @ Harlow, Essex (10miles)
49. August 10th: **Mynyddislwyn Mile** @ Newbridge, Monmouthshire, South Wales (1 mile).
50. August 12th: **Isle of Man Half Marathon** @ Ramsey, Isle of Man. (13.1 miles)
51. August 17th: **St Levan 10km** @ Penzance, Cornwall. (10km)
52. August 18th: **Race The Train** @ Twyn, Gwynedd. (14.7 miles).
53. August 26th: **Battle of Sedgemoor 10km** @ Langport, Somerset (10km)

SEPTEMBER

54. September 1st: **Braemar Highland Games** @ Braemar Castle, Royal Deeside. (3.3 miles)
55. September 2nd: **Great Scottish Run** @ Glasgow (13.1 miles)
56. September 8th: **Test Way Relay** @ Stockbridge, Hampshire. (5.7 miles).
57. September 9th: **The Grizzly** @ Seaton, Devon. (19.7 miles)
58. September 15th: **Round Norfolk Relay** @ King's Lynn, Norfolk. (16.6 miles)
59. September 22nd: **Sleepwalker Midnight Marathon** @ Talybont on Usk, Brecon, Powys, South Wales (20 miles)
60. September 27th: **Ron Hill Birthday 5km** @ Littleborough, Lancashire. (5km)
61. September 30th: **BUPA Great North Run** @ Newcastle, Tyneside. (13.1 miles)

OCTOBER

62. October 7th: **Chiquita Bananaman Chase** @ Milton Keynes, Buckinghamshire. (10km)
63. October 11th: **IRC Haslar 10km run** @ Gosport, Hampshire. (10km)
64. October 14th: **Swindon Half Marathon** @ Swindon, Wiltshire. (13.1 miles)
65. October 20th: **Bushy Park Time Trial** @ Hampton Court, Middlesex. (5km)
66. October 21st: **Stroud Half Marathon** @ Stroud, Gloucestershire. (13.1 miles)
67. October 28th: **BUPA Great South Run** @ Portsmouth, Hampshire. (10 miles)

NOVEMBER

68. November 4th: **Guy Fawkes 10** @ Ripley, North Yorkshire. (10 miles)
69. November 11h: **Grand Union Canal Half Marathon** @ Cowley, Middlesex. (13.1 miles)
70. November 17th: **Brampton to Carlisle Race** @ Carlisle, Cumbria. (10 miles)
71. November 18th: **Gill Pimblott Memorial 5km** @ Tyldesley, Manchester (5km).
72. November 25th: **Leeds Abbey Dash 10km** @ Leeds, Yorkshire. (10km)

DECEMBER

73. December 2nd: **Liverpool Santa Dash** @ Liverpool, Merseyside. (5km)
74. December 9th: **Keyworth Turkey Trot Half Marathon** @ Keyworth, Nottinghamshire. (13.1 miles)
75. December 16th: **Merthyr Mawr Christmas Pud** @ Merthyr Mawr, Glamorgan. (5.7 miles).
76. December 22nd: **Christmas Pudding Dash** @ Battle, East Sussex (5 miles).
77. December 26th: **Round the Lakes, Poole 10km** @ Poole, Dorset. (10km)
78. December 30th: **Maldon Mud Race** @ Maldon, Essex. (400 yards)
79. December 31st: **Nos Galan** @ Mountain Ash, Rhondda Valley. (5km)
80. **Bryan Clifton Memorial Midnight Run** @ Milford, Derbyshire. (2km).

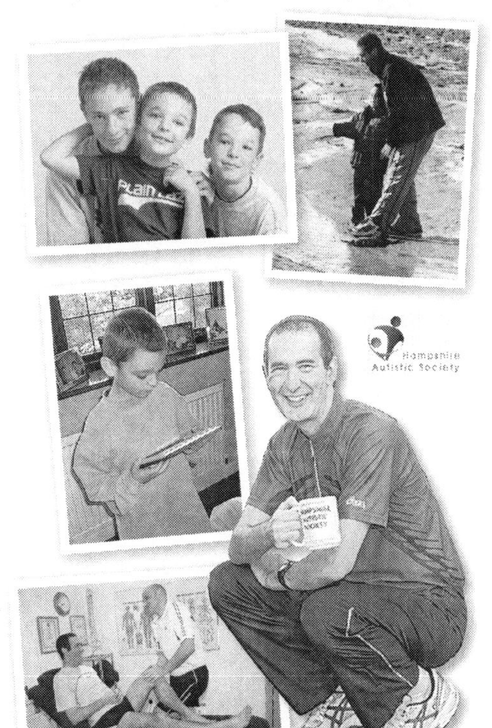

"The man who can drive himself further once the effort gets painful is the man who will win."

Introduction

DECEMBER 31st 2006

SO this is it. Milford, a village lying in the heart of Derbyshire's Derwent Valley, and the starting point for a year-long running adventure.

It's not the most picturesque or romantic of places to set out on this challenge. Given the choice I would much prefer a snowy peak in Scotland, a misty moor in Yorkshire, or perhaps a rural setting in the Cotswolds; one of those little chocolate box villages sprinkled with thatched cottages and the rich smell of wood smoke spilling out of the chimneys. Instead, I am celebrating New Year's Eve in this tiny hamlet which has the busy A6 between Duffield and Belper choking its way through.

Milford grabbed a name for itself during the Industrial Revolution when a string of textile mills sprung up alongside the River Derwent. Jedediah Strutt built a water-powered cotton mill, and after that the village took off big-time. Sadly, much of the 150-year-old mill building was demolished between 1952 and 1964. A huge chimney-stack now dominates the Milford skyline, while what remains of the old mill has been transformed into workshops. But hey, you've got to start somewhere.

It's New Year's Eve, 30 minutes to the witching hour, and Milford Social Club is a surreal location as a starting point for this adventure. This is a typical, old-fashioned Working Men's Club with a tatty, tired and worn feel to it. Several locals are sat round a table at one end of the room nursing pints and sharing a joke. Hazel, a lady in the autumn of her years, holds custody of the bar exchanging the latest village gossip with a Scottish lady perched on a stool, smoking away. "Help yourself to some food, duck," says Hazel, smiling and pointing to platefuls of pickled onions, sausage rolls and potato wedges. I bet the carbo-loading Kenyans don't get offered this sort of feast before a big race.

With the clock slowly ticking towards midnight, runners are streaming steadily into the social club where race organiser, David Denton, has taken up a position at the other end of the room. Sat next to the electronic one-arm bandit machine, David is scribbling down race entries while handing out numbers and safety pins. With his round spectacles and grey beard, David has that professorial look. He's an interesting guy who has been organising races for 40 years, yet spends the months commuting between homes in Derbyshire, Prague and India; a strange combination of holiday destinations.

New Year's Eve is a time to get well and truly bladdered. Usually in that hazy, drunken stupor, it is a chance to look back on the last 12 months with rose-tinted spectacles. Over a sherbert or two, it is an opportunity to agree that though it was another pile of trite, next year can only get better. It is not a time to throw on your running shoes, definitely not if you're sober. But on the pavement outside the Milford Social Club dozens of suspiciously sane souls, clad in tight leggings and fluorescent tops, plus the occasionally woolly hat, are limbering up for the Bryan Clifton Memorial Midnight Run which is held every New Year's Eve at three minutes to midnight.

I must be out of my skull for this, my first race in a 12-month running adventure. I intend to run into 2007 with this 2 kilometre dawdle beside the Derwent. The goal, injury and sanity permitting, is to be back here in Milford on December 31st next year to run out of 2007.

You will remember how the Queen had her 'annus horribilis'. Well, for the duration of my 'annus off-my-trolley-us', I have mapped out a schedule which even Alan Whicker would be proud of, criss-crossing the British Isles in pursuit of races of varying size, significance and distance - from distances as short as two kilometres to a gruelling 26-mile marathon. There will be the huge mass participation events such as the Great North Run, and smaller village races. For instance, I have entered the Round the Tree 3 in Torrington, North Devon, which runs shoulder to shoulder with a traditional May Day fete – Morris dancers and May pole at no extra charge!

There will be the historical events like the Blaydon Races on Tyneside, the Braemar Games in Scotland, which usually attracts the odd royal or two, and the Wenlock Olympian Games in Shropshire – an event stretching back more than a century and which was the inspiration behind the current moneybags Olympic extravaganza.

Throw in a few obscure races such as the Race the Train in North Wales, the Maldon Mud Race and Cani-X in Wiltshire, plus real toughies with names which give you the collywobbles by simply filling out the entry form – the Terminator, and the Grizzly – plus a varied programme which includes road running, fell running, cross country, orienteering, and hashing....and I'm already breathless at the thought of what lies ahead.

So, as I line up in Milford, with a light drizzle falling, the seeds of doubt are beginning to creep in. Why am I trying to keep warm in the damp East Midlands when I would much rather be seeing in the New Year with my family back home on the south coast?

Well, let me explain. With the advent of the new millennium, running and myself had become best pals. For years I had played Sunday league parks football. These were pub scraps which frequently got nasty, often involving some mouthy guys whose sole intention was to kick lumps out of you, to teach you a form of ball control which pitched your singing voice from a sturdy tenor to a schoolboy treble – and that was all in the dressing room before the game even got under way!

With a young family of three boys, and a busy working life as a sports journalist, I decided the time was right to hang up the football boots and put away the dubbin in order to spend more quality time with my family. At least with running, I figured, I could get up early on a Sunday morning for a canter along the cliffs near my home which overlooks the Solent and the Isle of Wight, yet still be home in time for breakfast.

That clever plan backfired big-time four years later, just before I was packing a suitcase to head up to the capital for the London Marathon. My then wife suddenly announced that she no longer wanted to be married; she was bored, desired independence and needed her own space – so how about a separation? What fantastic timing she had! Who needs pre-race pep talks with searing thunderbolts like that?!

So I may have helped to blow a marriage over my running, but I've been pretty faithful to running as a new love of my life. We've been together for more than 7,500 miles over six eventful years (yes, I am sad enough to keep a training diary for every time I've laced up a pair of running shoes). That, by my reckoning, is the equivalent of running from London to Honolulu – give or take a couple of hundred miles. If I had have known that sad anorak fact six years ago then I would have given up the wife, the nipple rash and the blisters, and settled for a one-way ticket to the Pacific in the hope of meeting a sassy, sexy female extra off Hawaii Five-O – "book 'em Dano!"

Instead I joined a running club, began to run four, sometimes five times a week, and enjoyed a modicum of success. Okay, so I have never won anything; come to think of it, I've never been anywhere near the top ten, although more runners have tended to finish behind me than ahead of me in races. I've competed in two London Marathons, the second time pipping the gorgeous model Nell McAndrew for a very respectable (and possibly never to be beaten) personal best time of 3 hours 19 minutes.

But it isn't the racing or the personal bests which does it for me. Nor is it the endorphins which hit you after each run, although they are cheaper than a couple of E's down the local spit and sawdust nightclub. It is the sheer pleasure of running; running free, running with others, drawn together by a common bond.

I love the camaraderie. I love the banter before, during and after the races. I love meeting the characters running in some truly spectacular settings. I love running in remote locations, revelling in the wilderness miles away from the nearest roads with only the sound of cow bells and the smell of cow dung to disturb the concentration. I also love taking part in the big races featuring thousands of runners where the wonderful support from the crowds makes you feel ten feet tall. Run the London Marathon, and if you are an atheist it is the closest you'll ever come to a spiritual experience.

Each race is a personal challenge, each packs its own adventure. With running, there is no time to stand still or get bored because if you do then you risk being passed by some grey-haired old geezer wearing Chariots of Fire style shorts. So in pursuit of doing something decidedly different, the idea for the challenge was born.

Tied in with this was a desire to promote the cause of autism, something which has affected me deeply through my nine-year-old son Ross, who is severely autistic. He has no communication, is still in nappies, and requires round-the-clock attention.

People with autism have a lifelong disability that interferes with their ability to interact with the world around them. The nature of the disability, first identified during the 1940's, means they can lack the range of skills essential for independent life in the outside world.

These skills are categorised into three main areas; social interaction, communication and imagination. People with autism will have problems in all three, but they will not necessarily have all of the problems.

With social interaction, they are unable to make friends outside of the family, appear aloof and indifferent to people, and tend to spend large amounts of their time alone.

Communication is another key indicator through lack of speech, difficulty with using symbols, a lack of eye contact and body language and an inability to understand common gestures or facial expressions.

And with imagination, there is an absence of imaginative activities of play with those outside the family. Those with autism have repetitive behaviour patterns and are resistant to any change of routine. They also have an obsession with particular objects.

Since Ross was diagnosed with autism at the age of four, I have studied the effects of autism closely, and have worked with the Hampshire Autistic Society who reckon that in that county alone there are 16,000 people with autism – a disability which touches the lives of half a million people nationally.

The cause is unknown, and a cure is not even on the radar. Autism is called a Spectrum Disorder because every individual will present with their own type and severity of their problems. Currently, autism affects about 50 in every 10,000 people.

A child with autism looks no different from any other child of his age – Ross has a face of an angel and to look at his picture you would not know he has this life-changing disability. This leads strangers to assume that the child is wilfully badly behaved. Or they blame the parents for not controlling the child.

So here I had a winning combination of running and autism, with a desire to use the challenge as a vehicle to promote awareness of autism wherever I visited in the UK.

For the past 15 months I have been mapping out races around the country which I thought would be fun, both to run and to write about. On the study wall back home in Southampton, I've plotted races with a deep history to them, races in parts of the British Isles where I have never visited, races whose very names have a tale to tell.

Running is full of colourful characters and interesting personalities for whom the simple act of putting one foot in front of the other, at a pace which sometimes teeters just above walking, is part of their life and culture. Each one of these figures has a story worth telling. If, for no-one else's interest other than my own, I wanted to convey this culture.

So on the pretext of doing a bit of sightseeing with a difference in 2007, here I am, on December 31st, warming up on the edge of the Peak District about to take part in the last race of 2006 in the UK and the first of 2007. Knowing my current racing speed, and with a start-time of 11.57pm, two kilometres is going to take me until almost five past midnight before crossing the finish line. Though for once, my finishing time is not important.

It is going to be the first of many finishes, and the first of many souvenir race mugs which I will collect along the way.

After all, you know what they say: running is a mug's game!

“Over the years, I’ve given myself a thousand reasons to keep running, but it always comes back to where it started. It comes down to self-satisfaction and a sense of achievement.”

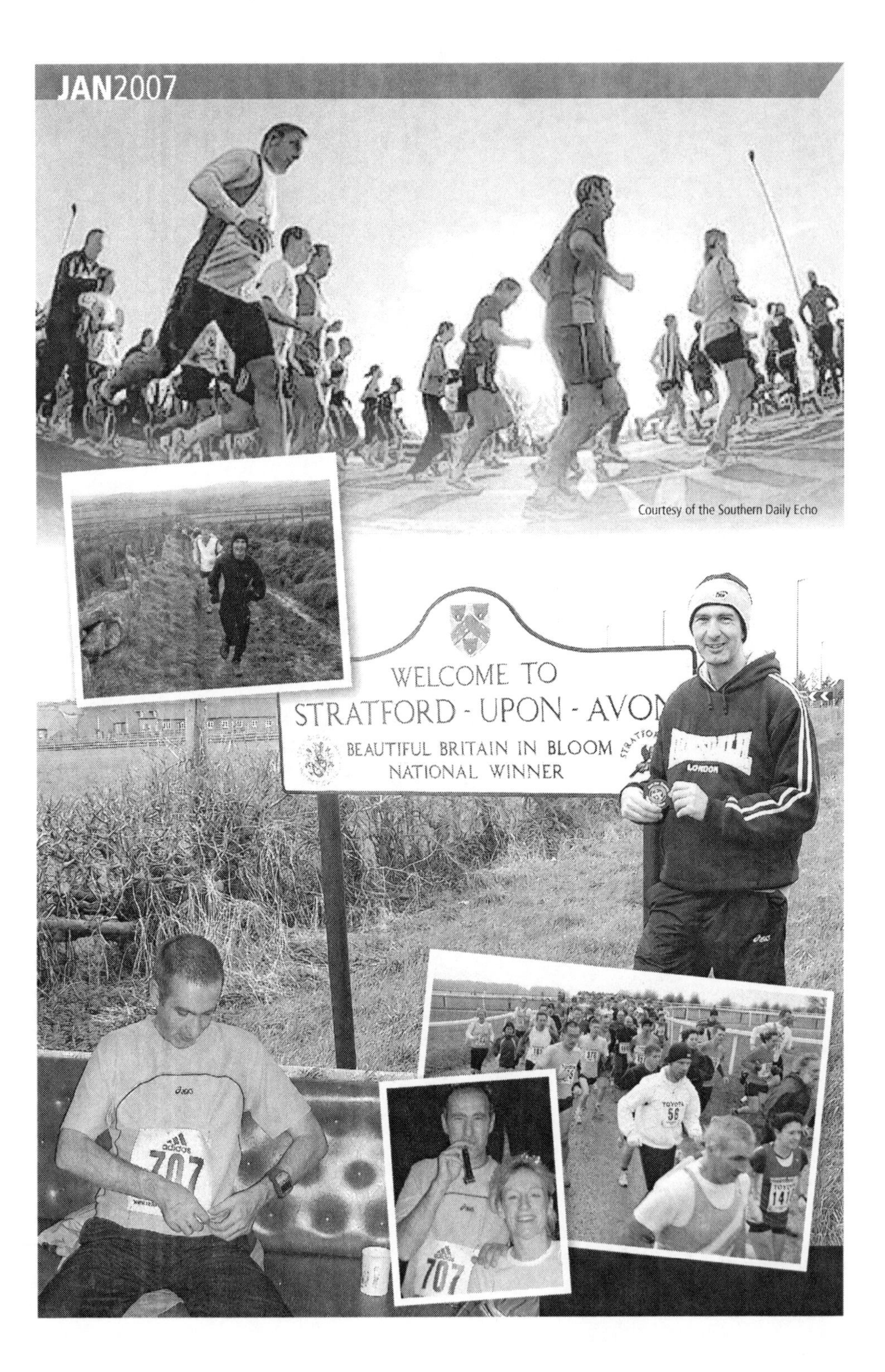

Courtesy of the Southern Daily Echo

JANUARY

1. Bryan Clifton Memorial Race @ Milford, Derbyshire.

WITH a straightforward and almost understated "Are you ready? Go!", my 12-month running adventure got under way in Milford at precisely 11.57pm on New Year's Eve, 2006.

No fanfare, no countdown, no loud klaxon – just four simple words began my journey around the British Isles.

Gathered on a wet street in Derbyshire for the Bryan Clifton Memorial Run, 50 of us had turned our backs on friends and families, deciding instead to see in the New Year in a sweaty and sober state. Bryan Clifton was the team manager of organiser David Denton's old club Tipton Harriers. He ran the first of the midnight races when it was held on December 31st, 1999, finishing 11th, and then dropped dead three minutes into this century. "Such a sad way to start a new millennium, but what a wonderful way to go," said David.

Among those taking part in the 2006 race was Fay, a lovely lady who lived in the nearby village of Cromford, which sits on the edge of the Peak District in Derbyshire. She had tried to persuade her family to come to the race, but they preferred to do the "Auld Lang Syne" bit in the comfort of their own home. "It would have been nice for the family to be here, but running is what I love doing. This will be a different start to the New Year," she insisted.

Fay, who had recently run the London Marathon in 4 hours 40 minutes, thrust a £2 coin in my palm when she heard I was raising money for autism. It was the first donation to the year-long fund-raising for the Hampshire Autistic Society, my chosen cause. "That's so wonderful, I wish I had time to do that," she offered enviously. "This year I did a triathlon for the first time which was fantastic. I never thought I would finish one, but why not? Even at my age!"

After wishing her a three-minute early "Happy New Year", I left my girlfriend Liz at the start line to run with Fay while I stretched and warmed up.

Liz had driven up with me from the south coast for this New Year's weekend. We had met at our running club, Stubbington Green Runners, a couple of years ago, and been living together for the past year. Two separated folk in their early forties wondering what lay ahead for them in the second part of our lives. We had got together and in that time Liz has been a source of huge encouragement towards my running project. She has helped dissect the awesome schedule, provided the occasional shoulder to cry on plus a kindly ear to listen to my frustrated tones – a patient lady who has been the perfect sounding board.

Liz was on chauffeuring duties for this first trip north of the campaign. I had fallen asleep in the passenger seat on our drive to the midlands on December 30th having been up since 3am. My job as deputy editor of the Southern Daily Echo in Southampton meant I always had my mobile phone by the side of my bed. So when the call came through at this ungodly hour that Saddam Hussein had just been executed in Baghdad some three hours before the presses rolled for the first edition, I was in the office within 20 minutes, re-writing and re-designing the first five pages of the newspaper, together with the chief sub-editor.

Besides photographic duties, Liz was great company to have around for this first weekend of running. A former Royal Navy nurse, and now a senior nurse looking after cancer patients at Southampton General Hospital, Liz reckoned that Fay was more her gentle pace as they set off together down the short, steep hill from the Milford Social Club and onto the A6 where the unusually quiet road was lit by the sombre glow of orange street lamps.

It was eerily tranquil along this straight road towards Duffield with barely any traffic passing as we made our way along the pavement through leaf-strewn puddles. The only sound was the noise of our footsteps. Then right on cue at midnight, the night sky was lit up by fireworks. It could have been choreographed, but it wasn't. From private fireworks displays around the valley, rockets exploded above us in a multitude of brilliant colours. Happy New Year – welcome to 2007.

At this moment I reached the turning bollard in Duffield, manned by a lone guy wearing a fluorescent yellow marshal's bib. I was struggling a little, breathing heavily. My legs felt leaden. I was passed by a few runners as we headed back towards Milford, the Christmas lights from the Strutt Arms on the edge of the village acting as our homing beacon. A few cars sped past, their horns blaring noisily in celebration, the now sporadic fireworks display providing a wonderful backdrop on a chilly and damp evening. Fortunately, despite a heavy shower an hour beforehand, the nasty stuff had held off in Derbyshire around midnight– all around the UK, storms had put paid to Hogmanay celebrations in Edinburgh and Glasgow, and prompted a string of New Year's Eve party cancellations elsewhere, including fireworks displays in Liverpool and Newcastle, plus an open air concert in Belfast.

Soon, the finish was in sight just off the A6, with a short, sharp rise up Chevin Road where I crossed the line to the sound the timekeeper shouting "nine-eighteen". A gentle 9 minutes and 18 seconds for 2km and 11th place – ironically the same placing as Bryan Clifton in the inaugural event. The winner of the first race of 2007 in the UK was Adam Rollitt from Ashbourne Running Club in a time of 7 minutes 22 seconds. Liz and Fay finished a couple of minutes behind me in 25th and 26th places, looking refreshed and pleased with their runs.

Back inside the warm trappings of the social club, the locals still hadn't moved from their trusted spot in the corner. Hazel and the Scottish lady were still gassing by the bar. Tea and toast was being served up for the runners who had ventured to Derbyshire from as far afield as Fife, Essex, Bath and Merseyside for an event which forms part of a weekend of races which David Denton puts on every New Year.

Liz and I smartly made our excuses from the social club, cutting a quick dash back to our hotel to catch a few hours' sleep before the next stage of this adventure.

2. Brown Willy 6 @ Bodmin Moor, Cornwall.

IT WAS a crazy plan – two races, eight miles in running distance, spread 280 miles apart - but at 4am, with little more than three hours' sleep, the alarm shattered our tender eardrums and within half an hour we had washed, changed, packed and checked out of our hotel room in Derbyshire before heading south. It was the fastest I had ever seen Liz move in the morning! Liz slept while I drove through the early hours on quiet motorways south carrying a few New Year stragglers back to their homes.

When I was planning this mad escapade, the initial idea had been to run in Derbyshire on New Year's Eve and then head north-east to take part in the Morpeth to Newcastle road race, which is one of Britain's oldest road races. Sadly, because of spiralling police costs and lack of a committed sponsor, the event, which celebrated its centenary in 2004, was scrapped in September 2006.

The four-and-a-half hour journey to Cornwall was broken up by a brief stop at the Gordano Services just off the M5 near Bristol for a breakfast of hot chocolate and almond croissants. It gave me time to come to terms with what I had just started. After months of thinking, planning and talking about it, this was the reality. I was tired, but excited. Milford had not been what I had expected, but it had provided the perfect, low-key start to 12 months of adventure. This was going to be a year of discovery.

A few hours later at just before 10am, we pulled off the A30 on to Bodmin Moor, and to our destination, the Jamaica Inn. The weather was glorious. It was a crisp and sunny New Year's Day, and already, an hour and a half before the race start, a posse of runners were mingling in the pub car park. More ominously, there was a Land Rover from Cornwall Search & Rescue stationed close by.

The origins of the Brown Willy 6 are about as hazy as the swirling mist on Bodmin Moor. However it was a man called Frank Squibb, well known within the Cornish running scene, who, a few years back, got together a group of friends for this out and back run on New Year's Day. Soon the group grew, and the run became more organised. Truro Running Club now put together the race with Richard Willson, the man at the helm. "Last year we had gale-force winds. I went out early to put up the signs, and they were flying all over the moor," Richard told me beforehand. "You're in for a treat. It's a run over some poor grazing land, then onto some open boggy, moorland, and a rocky last stretch to Brown Willy."

Jamaica Inn, the supposedly haunted old coaching inn which was made famous by Daphne du Maurier's novel of the same name, was steadily filling up. Here was a coaching inn built in the mid-eighteenth century and once used by weary travellers heading on the turnpike between Launceston and Bodmin having crossed the wild and dangerous moor. Some of the travellers were a little less respectable than most, using Jamaica Inn to hide away the contraband which had been smuggled ashore.

They're a good and lively crowd in Cornwall. "Aren't you the fella who's running round the British Isles?" asked one guy at the registration desk. "I saw the article in Runner's World." "Yeah, that's me," I replied and soon a crowd of folk were sharing tales about running in the Duchy, suggesting a few races which I should include in the project.

I managed to persuade Anna, one of the Truro Running Club crowd and who was out injured, to take my camera for a few shots. She was marshaling at a point high up on the moor. "You're going to find it tough," she warned. "Last year when we got to Brown Willy you couldn't stand up. The weather was that bad. We had to crawl around the tor."

Race time arrived, and by then the weather had clouded over. I was concerned what to wear, so I borrowed one of Liz's waterproof jackets, put on three layers of top clothes, added leggings, a woolly hat and donned a pair of gloves. The Michelin man takes on Brown Willy! Ultimately, my choice of clothing was to prove wise because during the race the weather closed in. Some of these hardy Cornish folk set out in nothing more than a vest and shorts – nutters! Liz had also decided to give the race a go latching onto a group of ladies in fancy dress from Newquay Running Club, one wearing a

Dalmatian outfit, another dressed as a cat, and a third carrying balloons to lift her up Brown Willy. They had been on the lash the night before, and reckoned that since Brown Willy would be hard, they might as well have some fun!

The first part of the moorland run was fairly steady as we made our way up a rough track, but very soon this race became a test of navigation when the ground became boggier and wetter. Trying to find the driest path was the key, leaping over ditches, stepping off stones to avoid the glutinous mud, while seeking out the slightly higher and drier ground. I managed to stick behind one lady runner who seemed to be picking the right dry and solid patches to run on. Others weren't so lucky, and Liz had one of her shoes sucked off by the mud which pulled at her ankles.

The Brown Willy 6 isn't so much a race, as a feat of endurance; the perfect hangover cure. On this day it was a great cobweb clearer running across the moorland with the wind picking up and the rain starting to fall. As the weather closed in, it soon became apparent how this was a race to dig in and survive. What was worrying was that even though we had been running for 20 minutes, I could not see Brown Willy.

Hail was now biting into my face and conditions were getting treacherous. Picking my way up a ridge, leapfrogging off stones in the middle of bogs, and trying to feel my way with mud-sodden shoes, I was honing in on anything resembling solid ground. Suddenly Brown Willy soared into view way off in the distance, its summit reaching to the sky.

No, that's not Brown Willy, I tried to convince myself, fearful of the ascent which lay ahead, surely that's Rough Tor, the other big hill on Bodmin Moor. Who was I trying to kid? The ant-like sight of runners picking their way up and down the sheer face of Brown Willy – at 1,293 feet the highest point in the Duchy – meant the only way was up.

There was no way you could run up Brown Willy. "Does anyone know where the chair lift is?" I wise-cracked to other runners. No-one laughed, no-one answered. Everyone was cream-crackered, pushing up off their knees along the side of this mini-mountain.

"Happy New Year" offered a wrapped up Richard Willson, standing near the summit. A few seconds later, Sherpa Tensing-like, I'd reached the tor – a stony collection of rocks at the top. On a clear day, you can see both Cornish coastlines from the peak. Today, the view was still spectacular, but the clouds had rolled in and my eyes roamed over the remote and bleak moor which was the route back to the finish.

The return to Jamaica Inn was painful and hard. Tiredness is a cruel enemy. Where once I was stepping off rocks and clearing ditches, now my aching legs could only claw their way through the mud. "How do you eat an elephant? - one piece at a time," goes the expression. When I am feeling drained and up against it on a run, that's the mantra which rings in my head. Runners were steering their way past my weary body, including one slip of a lad from Cornwall Running Club with all the energy and dexterity of a mountain goat! For me this was a battle of pure attrition.

Sixty six minutes and 6.8 miles after leaving Jamaica Inn, I was back home which was when the heavens really opened, and the rain pounded down. "This is what we call Cornish sunshine," quipped one orange-bibbed marshal, hiding under an umbrella in the car park. "Guaranteed sunshine, all year round!"

The winner, David Roper, had finished 20 minutes ahead of me. I was exhausted, I was soaked, but thrilled at having finished. Liz eased up the final hill half an hour later delighted to have survived the experience. "What a way to start the New Year," she said, red-faced and her blonde hair sodden with rain and sweat. We collected our race memento, a framed picture of Brown Willy, which I plan to turn into a dartboard.

Running two races in less than 12 hours spread 280 miles apart was always going to be a tough ask. But as the launching pad to a year of racing around the British Isles it was the perfect appetiser.

3. Tadworth 10 @ Tadworth, Surrey.

BACK HOME in Southampton for the first week of 2007, I was getting some alarming knee pain. This was clearly the result of the punishing hill run in Cornwall, particularly the descent when my knees took quite a pounding.

Since the autumn, I had been seeing a sports physiotherapist on a fortnightly basis. Mark Diment is one of life's characters. Folically-challenged, he's the spitting image of the comedian Lee Hurst, who made his name on the TV panel game "They Think It's All Over". A young guy in his 30s, Mark is funny, great company and even when he's contorting your body all over the place, the guy has always got a wisecrack up his sleeve. What's more, he's good. Mark was my insurance and a good investment too. One major injury at any time this year and the whole project would have been scuppered.

What was worrying me most was the next four months leading up to the London Marathon in April when I would be running long distances, both in races and in training, putting my body under enormous stress when the potential for injury was at its greatest.

Running is punishing, especially on the joints. With every strike of the ground your feet absorb three to four times your body weight. If only it was possible to surgically implant a few extra shock absorbers in the legs to get me through the crunching demands of running.

So when I went to see Mark a few days after the two New Year races he assured me there was no major damage to the knees. Mark is a strong guy with firm hands which grip vice-like into your muscles. He went to work on the hamstrings, quadriceps, as well as my back. I felt good, I felt partially reassured, though in the back of my mind was that nagging worry about whether my body would hold up – and there were still 78 races to go!

As a result I quickly decided to change the schedule and abandoned the idea of competing in the Hampshire Cross Country Championships in Basingstoke. It was too risky, especially with a race the following day in Surrey.

Tattenham Corner is a name revered across the sporting world. This fearsome, sloping turn at the top of the Epsom Downs has provided the backdrop to many exciting finishes to The Derby. Named after a manor house which mysteriously disappeared, Tattenham Corner is a tricky hairpin turn with a sharp downhill drop of about 100 feet some five furlongs from the finish.

Many famous horses and their jockeys have turned on the magic at this iconic sporting landmark. Lester Piggott on Nijinsky in 1970, Geoff Lewis with Mill Reef a year later, and Sea Bird who, in 1965, was sixth going into Tattenham Corner when jockey Pat Glennon stepped on the gas to produce an astonishing victory. More notoriously, it was the spot where, in 1913, the suffragette Emily Davison was killed when she threw herself at the King's horse, Anmer.

Well let's add another memorable sporting moment to that glorious yet notorious list, for Tattenham Corner was the scene in early January 2007 where, despite driving rain and a fierce wind blowing off the North Downs, I performed a running striptease! The event was the Tadworth 10, a 10-mile running race which attracted more than 700 competitors on two loops, starting and finishing at Epsom racecourse.

When I arrived at the course with my father as company, it was blowing a hooley. Conditions were not pleasant as most competitors sought sanctuary in their cars before the race. Like a teenage girl sitting excitedly in her bedroom before going out on a date, I couldn't decide what to wear! The car was my bedroom. My dad and I sat inside a vehicle which was rapidly steaming up while I pulled various garments out of my sports bag. I threw on several top layers, some thigh-length shorts to protect the hamstrings, and a woolly hat to complete the garish-looking green outfit.

What a mistake! First off, no-one would run anywhere near me because I was visually polluting the race. And secondly, within a mile I was sweating like a weight-watcher in a cake shop. Not only did I look bad, I was smelling pretty rank too.

The race took runners up an energy-sapping hill into the village of Tadworth, and then meandered back towards the racecourse.

I started steadily, but soon realised a mile or two in that I was overheating. At Tattenham Corner on the first of two five-mile circuits, I spotted my dad. I signalled him to put his camera away as I veered off course and headed in his direction taking my clothes off. Other runners looked at me with a mixture of confusion and bewilderment. I was half naked by the time I reached my embarrassed father, threw him my clothes, pulled on a skimpy running vest and headed on. What a relief, I felt liberated!

The race itself was uneventful and soulless. The marshals were great and encouraging, the course was challenging, but there was very little race atmosphere. It was muddy and testing. I ran part of the way with Philip, who lived nearby in Elmbridge and had taken up running in the past year. He reckoned the sport had also taken two inches off his waistline. "Running's become part of my life," he said. Ironically, after all that stripping, the race memento was a piece of clothing – the dinkiest pair of racing gloves you have ever seen in your life, small enough to probably only fit a child.

The week after the race, though, I felt dreadful. Not only was injury the greatest opponent to this challenge, but so was illness. Going to see the physiotherapist every fortnight was like a two-weekly service for my car at the garage – and a darn sight cheaper. Since before Christmas, I had also been writing a food diary to make sure that I was eating and drinking the right stuff, as well as getting a proper balance of nutrition.

Then just before Christmas, after all the publicity about flu jabs, I decided to get one myself. Working in a hospital, Liz and the rest of the nursing staff receive free flu jabs annually. I thought of dressing up and posing as one of Liz's team, but her nurse's uniform, which is an unsexy mauve colour and looks like something a cardinal would wear in church, wouldn't fit. So I paid my £18 over the counter at one of those back-packing shops which, besides offering jabs to cover Japanese encephalitis, typhoid, yellow fever and hepatitis, also dispenses the flu vaccine.

But did it work? Did it heck! The week after Tadworth I felt like Babyshambles' Pete Docherty after a hard night's partying and carrying a voice which sounded like Bonnie Tyler at full pelt.

I tried to get a doctor's appointment, but the MI5 trained receptionist said they didn't have any appointments until later in the week. I called Liz and croaked my story. "Oh, tell them you've got a chest complaint. You're aching a bit, aren't you? That'll do the trick," she suggested.

Back to the surgery, patched through via GCHQ, I threw in a bit of acting straight out of the Kenneth Williams/Terry Scott School of Milking It, and the answer came back: "Can you get here in half an hour, Mr King?" "I'll try," I replied mournfully. The doctor said it was flu – plenty of rest, drink what you can and take paracetamol. I told him about the flu jab, he replied that this was no guarantee, in fact there was a pretty virulent strain doing the rounds which was why they were so busy. In a word, you could sense he was saying: "Why are you bothering me with this rubbish? Get out of my surgery so I can deal with some really ill, people who don't hoodwink my military-trained receptionists that they're about to have a heart attack."

4. Stubbington Green 10km @ Stubbington, Hampshire.

FEELING worse for wear through illness, it was a stroke of luck that I wasn't running the following weekend because event four was the Stubbington Green 10km. The race is organised by my club, Stubbington Green Runners, based around this small, but neat village which lies beside by the Solent.

Gary Littlecott was the race director. We've been good mates and training partners for a few years – never run downwind of Gazza because the man is a bottom burping nightmare; five years of running with him on a Sunday morning taught me this. He's the only runner I know who ought to be fitted with a catheter since he needs to go to the loo that often when we're out for a jog. No longer do we decide on running routes for their scenery along the coastline, but like a pair of boozers picking out hostelries for a pub crawl, we have to scour a map to decide how many public conveniences we will pass.

But he's a bloody good mate and so when a year earlier, in a brazen act of stupidity, he decided to take on the race director's role for the Stubbington Green 10k well, you know what they say about a friend in need...put your mobile on silent!

To be fair, Gary had the whole thing pretty well sussed. He had to, because although this prestigious road race has been going for donkey's years, it had tended to be run on a bit of a wing and a prayer. In this "no win, no fee", "there's no such thing as an accident" 21st century blame culture, the race desperately needed bringing up to date. Gary had to strip bare the event organisation. Possibly because I am a bit lippier than him, I tended to front up the meetings with the police, local council, highways authorities and traders. Trying to lay on a safe race for 1,000 runners on a six-mile route around the streets of Stubbington was no cake-walk. I came out of one meeting with the police distinctly troubled when they warned how messy things could get if you hadn't planned the event properly and got it badly wrong. So courses were re-measured, fresh risk assessments made, we decided to drop the wheelchair race simply because we could not safely run that event. We dallied with the idea of introducing chip timing - but that proved too costly. We cheesed off

Stubbington's traders by deciding to apply for a three-hour closure of the village square, and basically re-wrote the whole race plan.

Organising the Stubbington 10k was an agonising, waking up in the middle of the night in a sweat process, and I wasn't the one to shoulder the bulk of the burden. What would happen if a helicopter crashed on the road outside HMS Daedalus, which is where the Solent Coastguard is based? How would we cope with three foot of January snow on the morning of the race? Where are the mugs and trophies, and have we got enough portable loos – well, enough for Gary! Finally, the day came to pass. As part of my running adventure, this was one race I was not going to take part in. Gary would have killed me had I not been there to help. Instead, I arrived at day crack to begin the 101 jobs which needed sorting before the 10am start.

It wasn't quite Challenge Anneka because with the best laid plans we knew what we were doing. It was remarkable to see the village rapidly transformed into a running arena, and soon filled with several thousand people. I took myself to marshal at one of the critical points of the course where runners had to cross a busy road and head down a country lane near Lee-on-the-Solent Golf Course. Thankfully two police officers were on hand to help, and without any incident we got the runners safely through.

Sadly, the day wasn't totally incident-free. One runner was clipped on the legs by a car's trailer. Fortunately he did not require hospital treatment and went home with just a few grazes. Another motorist had a stand up row with the police and a marshal after he ignored a plea to stop and wait at a junction. Instead the imbecile edged his car past a crowd of runners. The marshal chased after him, banged his hand on the car bonnet and that was it! Despite the ample signage put up a week before, more than 20 police officers and special constables on duty, dozens of marshals lining the route, you still got some drivers who were impatient, wouldn't think, and risked causing accidents. They were just inconsiderate eggheads.

Despite this, the reaction from runners was very positive with just a few expressing concerns over the congested start. Among the stream of e-mails which followed the race, unbelievably we had one complaint that the water stations were positioned on the wrong side of the road. "Most runners are right-handed, so why on earth put in on the left-hand side and make it even harder?!" Almost as if in reply, another kind runner wrote: "Only a genius at pedantry could find fault with this race." – I rest my case!

5. Brass Monkey Half Marathon @ York.

THERE are certain types of runner who deserve the bargepole treatment. There are the Pepe Le Phews, the skunk-like scarecrows who give off an aroma which, if bottled, could be used as chemical warfare on a battlefield. Mixed with sweat, these lepers of the running community take body odour to a new, nauseating level.

Then there are the phlegm merchants who belong to two distinct categories – the dribblers and the gobbers. They are unsightly and uncouth, and it is advisable not to run downwind for fear of being afflicted by phlegm fall-out.

Finally, there are the heavy breathers who also fall into two groups. There are the "chuffer chuffers", a band of brothers and sisters who steam along in a race rasping like the Flying Scotsman. With every step they take, they chuff.

Their close cousins are the Meg Ryans – as in the infamous deli scene in the film "When Harry Met Sally" when Sally Albright (Meg Ryan) demonstrates how a woman can easily fool a man by a fake orgasm. Back on the road, there's no faking these running stunts. Put bluntly, with every breath they take it's as if they're having an orgasm. The only difference is that this gasping orgasm can last for over an hour – which, from my experience, is something you don't hear too often!

I had the misfortune to run with a Meg Ryan character at the Brass Monkey Half Marathon in York. The unfortunate lady came from one of the Leeds clubs, and as the race headed out from York Racecourse on a long, flat road through the picturesque village of Bishopthorpe, Meg was going stride for stride with the pack of runners.

Others looked around wondering what was going on. Having encountered this classic type of Meg in previous races, there was only one thing for it – step up the pace and lose her.

Easing away from the pack, I could hear her having orgasms in the distance as I latched onto a runner from the wonderfully-titled Idle Athletic Club. "What a great name for a club," I said. "Yeah, we're based Bradford way," replied the fella in the white and black singlet. "What's better is that there is an Idle Working Men's Club in the town. Classic!"

Mr Idle was good company. We were moving at quite a lick at seven-minute mile pace for this popular race, which is organised by Knavemire Harriers. Sadly, you don't see anything of historic York and the fabulous Minster since the run takes you right into the countryside. The course is as flat as the Fens, heading south to Bishopthorpe, onto Whinny Hills and back to the racecourse via Bishopthorpe.

Despite the Brass Monkey tag, the weather this year was kind. The showers held off, and although the wind picked up at times, it wasn't too chilly. This is reckoned to be one of the best half marathons in the country, and entries were sold out within a week of them opening the previous September. I wouldn't say this was the best, but the post-race sweatshirt was one of the better mementos.

The guy from Idle AC stuck with me on a loop which took in the picturesque villages of Appleton Roebuck and Acaster Malbis, before he'd had enough of my pedestrian pace and headed off into the distance. No sooner had he gone than Leeds's answer to Meg Ryan was back on my shoulder. I tried to press on, dodging the huge muddy puddles which littered the country lanes, but I simply couldn't lose her. Her wailing was doing my head in. You couldn't concentrate. Subconsciously, you altered the cadence of your footsteps to fit rhythmically in time with the Richter scale breathing. There was only one thing for it – I slowed down and let Meg Ryan inflict her Oscar-winning performance on someone else so I could enjoy the last few miles in peace.

Sympathetic to my plight, I mentioned the Meg Ryan story to my colleagues in the newsroom at the Southern Daily Echo, and a few days later when I arrived at work there was a gift lying on my desk. It was a noisy key ring which emitted the rising strain of a woman experiencing the heights of pleasure – clearly she must have been doing the washing up!

Liz ran finishing half an hour behind me having a great time with a group of lady runners from Dragons' Running Club, also from Leeds. They were gassing all the way, encouraging each other. Now that's what's running is all about.

Dramatically, the race was coated with intrigue. There were problems with the results because of number swapping, and even worse, there were allegations of cheating with reports of a couple of runners cutting off part of the loop and re-joining the race. I had seen one guy emerge from some bushes half way through the run, but had assumed he was having a quick constitutional. This was clearly a case for Inspector Morse.

All this reminded me of much-to-be-admired story of Fika and Sergio Motsoeneng who took part in the gruelling 90km Comrades Marathon in South Africa in 1999. Though not twins, there was a strong resemblance between the brothers who hatched a plan to run the race as a relay, exchanging places at toilet stops, and aided by car lifts at various stages. Sergio crossed the finish line in ninth place which came as a surprise to other runners who couldn't recall being overtaken. However, the brothers were exposed as cheats when television footage revealed they were wearing watches on different arms! Classic!

6. Not The Roman IX @ Stratford-upon-Avon.

A WEEK later, I had ventured from historic York to William Shakespeare's Stratford-upon-Avon where, not since the Montagues and Capulets were slugging it out, has there been so much argy-bargy in this sleepy Warwickshire town. It was here, of course, that Billy boy was born in 1564: and after rattling out a few good tales while living in London, he retired to his birthplace and lived in this Warwickshire town until his death in 1616.

Stratford-upon-Avon is a living legacy to William Shakespeare. In fact, there can be few towns that are dominated as much by one man. A town of culture, refinement, decorum? Don't you believe it! Because in one part of the town, the local athletics club has been having a right old ding dong with residents.

Every year, Stratford-upon-Avon Athletic Club stages the Not the Roman IX road race. This is a 12km run which starts and finishes at the National Farmer's Union Sports & Social Club. Three years ago the race almost folded. The locals weren't very happy with runners converging on them on a Sunday morning. Maybe it was the gaudy sight of all that lycra, the potent smell of Deep Heat lingering in the air, or possibly they didn't want to have their bacon and eggs disturbed by the sound outside their front drives of runners jogging up and down the street. "They were unbelievable moaning minnies," explained one lady as we were doing those old fashioned star jumps as a pre-race warm-up. "For just one morning a year, they didn't want all the noise and traffic. It was pathetic."

Now, as you drive towards the start of the race along the River Avon, there are some spectacular homes which smell of money. Knowing the tempestuous background to the race, I was half expecting to find a load of Lord Snooty's lining the start of the race holding placards and sounding hunting horns. But far from it. The houses near the race start consisted of a rag-tag of fairly ordinary, 1960s semi-detached homes. In the pre-race instructions, we had been warned to "avoid any arguments with local residents and refrain from using improper language". Runners were also instructed not to let any family or friends use the children's playground... "which was provided for local children only." What a fuss! Have you heard of anything so pompous or ridiculous?!

The race itself was a corker. Twelve kilometres, or about seven-and-a-half miles, out in the spectacular Warwickshire countryside. The one drawback was that the race route didn't take in the wonderful backdrop of Stratford itself. It was the same as at York the previous week. Such are the high police costs and logistics of staging a city centre run, that this is nigh on impossible. Instead we were treated to a superb saunter around the lanes around Stratford-upon-Avon, with a few testing climbs, including the imaginatively named Long Hill, followed by a spectacular downhill run through the pretty village of Loxley with a sharp hairpin bend thrown in for good measure. Apparently Loxley is an alleged burial ground of Robin Hood, with its rewarding views over Stratford and Shakespeare country.

To warn oncoming traffic along the route, the marshals carried these huge red flags which would have looked more at home in an old Soviet communist parade, rather than a race around country lanes in the middle of England! The run-in to the finish passed the rebellious residents. A few stood on their doorsteps watching us without expression. There was even a policeman patrolling the pavement to keep order. I waved at one elderly couple, offering a plaintive cry of "mornin'", but they didn't seem to want to know.

It didn't matter. A good race with a good atmosphere, I got a cracking time of 52 minutes for 92nd place, which I celebrated with a juicy hamburger and fries afterwards!

"Every morning in Africa a gazelle wakes up. It knows it must move faster than the lion or it will not survive. Every morning a lion wakes up and it knows it must move faster than the slowest gazelle or it will starve. It doesn't matter if you are the lion or the gazelle, when the sun comes up, you better be moving."

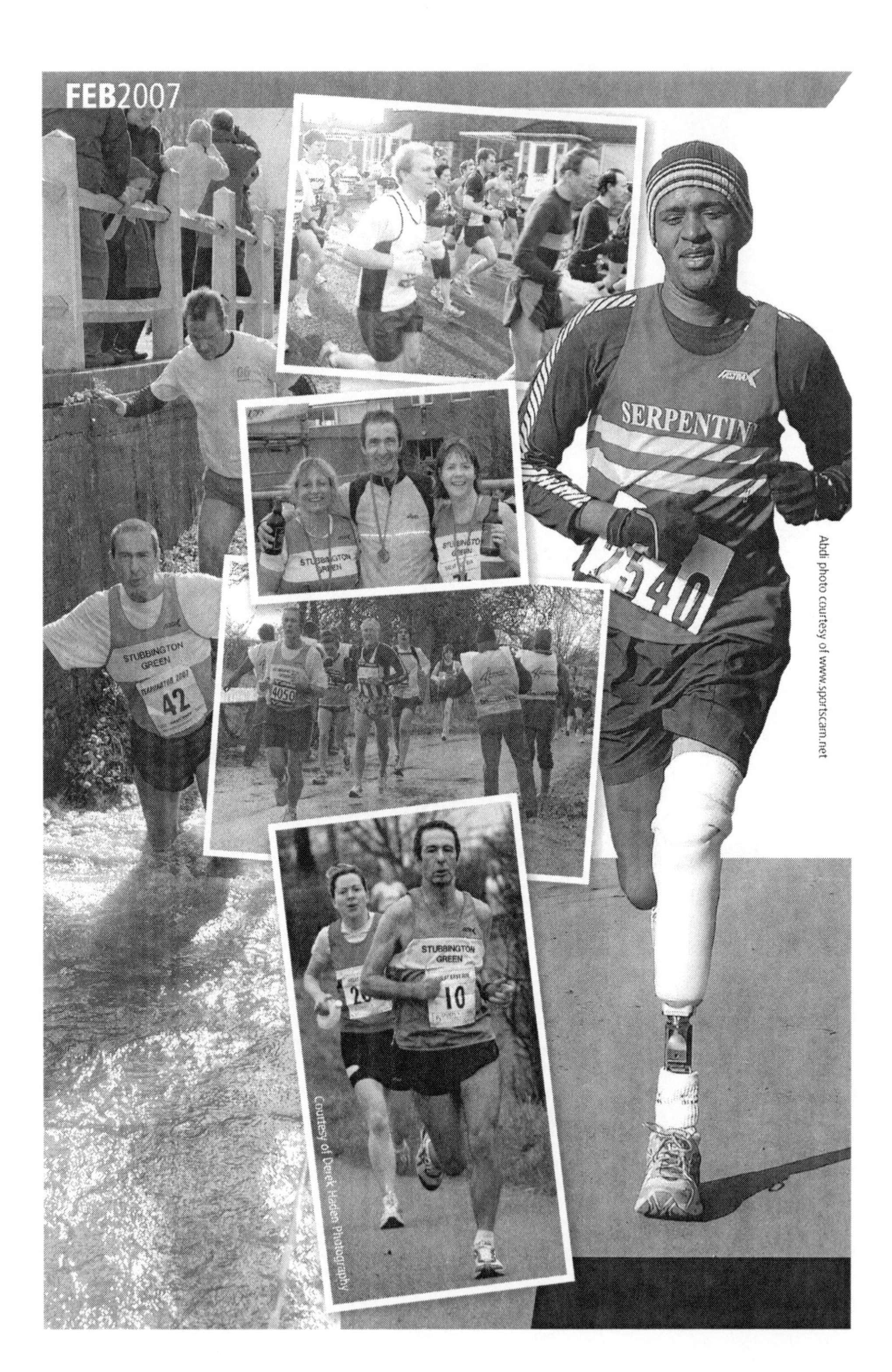

Abdi photo courtesy of www.sportscam.net

Courtesy of Derek Haden Photography

FEBRUARY

7. Watford Half Marathon @ Watford, Hertfordshire.

ABDIFATAH Dhuhulow was one of the victims of the civil war in Somalia – a country ravaged by famine and great suffering. In 1991, the African country was in turmoil following the collapse of Siad Barre's regime. Civil war erupted as an assortment of clan-based military factions competed for control.

Like the hundreds of thousands of other Somalis whose focus was simply staying alive and looking forward to tomorrow, Abdi, then just 10-years-old, found himself caught in the crossfire. "It was a terrible time for all of us, for all of my family," he recalled. "One day we were forced to flee the town where we were living. There were gunmen shooting everywhere. It was very frightening.

"I was hit by a bullet to my ankle which caused me to fall off the truck we were trying to get away on. As I fell off my left foot went under the wheel. Every bone was smashed. I wasn't able to get proper treatment at the time because of the situation in Somalia. There were no medical services so the bones healed incorrectly."

In 1998, Abdi came to the UK and a year later he had the first of five operations on his leg. But doctors were unable to save it, and in 2004 the decision was made to amputate Abdi's left leg. For many, especially those leading an active life as Abdi had before the accident, that would have been like a death sentence.

Instead, it offered him a new lease of life. He explained: "The physiotherapist at the hospital in London encouraged me to try running. Four months after the operation I had a go. I didn't know how to run with the prosthetic, so my physio taught me how to run around the park. It was very difficult because I had not used those muscles for a very long time, and at first I was in a lot of pain because I was putting so much weight on my good leg."

In time, Abdi gained confidence learning how to run by lifting the prosthetic and striking the ground correctly. Living in Fulham, he joined

Serpentine Running Club – one of the biggest running clubs in the country whose pillar box red and gold running vests are a familiar feature of running races the length and breadth of the country. While training with the club at Battersea Park, Abdi disguised the disability from other runners by wearing tracksuit bottoms. No-one had any idea he was an amputee, as he more than held his own at club sessions. Eventually, the secret was revealed to the amazement of his club-mates, and now the 26-year-old hasn't looked back since discovering the joys of running.

I caught up with Abdi in Hertfordshire early in February for the Watford Half Marathon, organised by Watford Harriers. The prosthetic looked impressive, though at the time he was about to swap that for a more modern one with skin cushioning, and probably go-faster stripes!

I was running well, using the event to build up important mileage towards the London Marathon which was in little more than two-and-a-half months time. A few miles from the finish I spotted Abdi looking pretty effortless in his running as others around him seemed to be struggling to hold the pace. Apart from being dumbstruck at seeing an amputee moving at such a pace, I was trying hard to close on him. But he was having none of this and as we entered Cassiobury Park for a final loop, Abdi was off and away to finish in a time of 1 hour 34 minutes 42 seconds, just 20 seconds ahead of me. It was the first time I have ever been beaten in a sprint finish by an amputee!

"Running is the best thing I have ever done," said Abdi afterwards. "When you have had such a bad time in your life you bottle it up, so running has enabled me to release the strain and feel relaxed."

Without wishing to patronise Abdi, you could not help but feel inspired by a man who insists he doesn't want to sell himself short in life, who gets on with life and enjoys it to the full. His troubles put our own lives into perspective by highlighting how trivial our simple travails are.

If you want tedious trivial travails, then one of the hottest potatoes dominating pre-race chatter was, would you believe, whether runners should or should not be allowed to wear iPods in races. It was almost anal in its subject matter, but one which was getting folk hot and bothered because of the number of accidents these mini musical beat boxes were causing. In their race instruction leaflets, some organisers were even advising competitors not to wear iPods or MP3 players, or face disqualification!

At Watford, for the first time, I decided to race with an iPod. Well, why not? When racing, you tend to be concentrating hard; keeping an eye on the watch and your pace, aware of runners around you, judging how fresh or laboured they are by listening to their breathing, and trying to work your way between packs.

However, with headphones on, and Frankie Goes To Hollywood blaring out, you're in a musical cocoon. Music can be inspirational, it can provide a focus, and for the Watford Half Marathon I wondered whether it would help take my mind off tired and aching limbs, particularly when I was likely to be struggling in the closing stages of the race.

As we lined up for the start in leafy Cassiobury Park, I was fairly pumped up. Music playing, I was oblivious to the atmosphere around me and shot off like an express train. I ran the first two miles in a suicidal for me 13 minutes. When the "Theme from Rocky" came on I swaggered down a country lane and threw a quick combination of a left jab and a right hook - Sly Stallone would have been proud of the neat footwork and deft flurry of fists. Some of my fellow competitors looked on at this strange fellow with the headphones.

But by the time Atomic Kitten came wafting through the iPod followed by Girls Aloud – okay, my taste in music has never been that cool – I struggled exhausted up the first of five pretty tough hills.

The music became an annoying distraction. I wasn't aware of those around me. I lost comprehension of pace, and a couple of times stepped into the path of other runners who replied with wise words which luckily I couldn't hear!

It was an experiment which went to pot, and by ten miles the headphones were starting to smart on my Mr Spock ears so I took them off. That's when I spotted Abdi and tried to sit in on the man's pace, but to no avail.

8. Stamford Striders' St Valentine 30km @ Stamford, Lincolnshire.

ABDIFATAH Dhuhulow's world couldn't be more different from the hard-as-nails character, Mary Picksley, who I met a week later in Stamford.

They certainly breed them tough up north! Mary is a slight lady, little more than 5 feet 5 inches tall in trainers and, put politely, in the autumn of her running years. In fact, I'm not sure quite how old she is, but the Yorkshire lass, who runs for the Steel City Striders Club in Sheffield, qualifies in the Veteran 55 age category.

Fifteen years ago at the London Marathon, Mary finished third in the veteran's category with a very respectable time of 3 hour 6 minutes which equates to a mile every seven minutes and six seconds. Now that is bloomin' good running.

If you want speed dating without the romance, because who in their right mind is going to find a red-faced, sweaty and out-of-breath runner dressed in shorts and a gaudy coloured top an attractive proposition, then running provides an interesting and very different proposition. After all, you're thrown together with a group of people who you probably haven't met before. This is a chance meeting with folk sharing a common interest drawn from a variety of backgrounds. The tiniest details are exchanged; "hi, I'm Pete, where the hell is Stubbington?"is often an opening gambit. You tend to strike up a bond, grabbing snatches of conversation and titbits about each other's lives. During the race you offer encouragement, help one-time strangers through the bad patches, make sure the other has got a drink from the water station, share Jelly Babies and energy-inducing gels before shaking hands at the finish funnel, unlikely ever to meet up again!

I would see Mary again later that April at the London Marathon – her 40th marathon – and we would be in touch several times during the course of the year, yet running with her in early February was typical of how these fast friendships are formed on the course. After the initial jockeying for position over the first couple of miles, we soon realised we were running close to each other's pace and, with only the briefest chatter, settled in together for the long run ahead.

"Will London be your last marathon?" I asked Mary, as we passed a water station, grabbing hold of a plastic cup from one of the young stewards. "No way," she replied. "I'll go on running marathons as long as I can keep running them. I never get tired of marathons, I never get tired of running. You know what's great about running? – you can eat what you like in the main, and you stay healthy."

The Stamford Striders' St Valentine's 30km race started by a school in Stamford, an attractive market town noted for its unspoilt Georgian streets and squares, its cluster of outstanding churches, and once the home of Daniel Lambert who earned the odd crust more than 200 years ago through his notoriety as the world's heaviest man. When Daniel died in 1809, he apparently weighed nearly 53 stone!! But I digress.

Now with Lincolnshire sitting so close to the pancake flat Fens of Cambridgeshire, where the nearest hillock eastwards is the Urals, I had expected the St Valentine's event to be a bit of a love-in; a gentle and steady run out. But no, the St Valentine's 30km race passed through four counties – Lincolnshire, Cambridgeshire, Rutland and Leicestershire, and seemed to produce a hill around every corner.

The race had an inauspicious start when a motorist, attempting to squeeze his way past almost 700 runners warming up, tried an audacious three-point turn. That livened things up, and delayed the start!

Mary was my pacer for most of the race. Despite her fragile frame, she was a terrier up the hills maintaining quite a ferocious pace. I spotted one chap early on who was running close to my race pace, but was put off by his sunflower shorts. That was a blind date I was going to dip out on. I later found out that his name was Russell Devitt from Shaftesbury Runners in London – named and shamed and our paths would cross again in Harlow six months' later when he was still sporting the offending attire. Russell eventually finished just ahead of me, but I knew I couldn't handle two and a half hours of being subjected to such an horrific visual assault. Call the fashion police, please!

So it was Metronomic Mary and me. We didn't talk much, except when I fell off the pace she would look behind and chivvy me along. She was almost metronomic in her running as we went through the miles at an even pace of seven and a half minutes.

The course was challenging, but it made for a great race. By one of the heart shaped distance markers placed on the kerb with just 4km left, Mary kicked on, and I couldn't respond. She eased past runners half her age and surged towards the finish. I managed a pleasing 2 hours 21 minutes, a couple of minutes down on Mary who was there to greet me at the end.

9. Great East Run @ Bungay, Suffolk.

IN THE early days, this mad-cap project had the working title of "Running For Trout". This was because one of the races I had targeted is called the Wincle Trout Run. The race takes place in the village of Wincle, near Macclesfield in Cheshire, every June. It is a 9 kilometre fell run which crosses woodlands, a river and high moorland, with 950 feet of climbing in the picturesque Dane Valley. What makes the race so novel is that every finisher receives a freshly-caught trout. It makes a change from the usual tacky medal or tatty t-shirt with ropey print which fades after the first few washes. When I initially contacted the organisers in Cheshire about the book idea they were delighted to hear I was coming. Sadly, the date of the Wincle Trout Run clashed with another race which suddenly crept into the schedule so that was when the book title changed.

However running the trout a close second in the unusual race souvenir stakes would be the bottle of beer I picked up at the Great East Run in Bungay, Suffolk. Elgood's Black Dog is a traditional dark mild which, according to the label, is full of roast malt flavour and brewed with the finest malt and hops, so it says on the label. What a shame I'm teetotal!

As race goodies go the Great East Run, which is held in the middle of February, is darn good. On the conveyer belt at the end of the race there was a bottle of beer, a small towel and a medal, plus assorted food snacks collected together in a snazzy drawstring bag. This was collected all this from a volunteer standing next to a couple of ladies serving steaming cups of tomato and golden vegetable soup. On a bitterly cold day it was perfect!

The Great North and the Great South runs are always huge mass participation events which are a launching pad for many people to exercise, as well as raising millions of pounds for charity. They are quite costly to enter too. However, the Great East Run has nothing to do with Nova International, organisers of the Newcastle and Portsmouth races. This 20km run in the Suffolk countryside is hosted by the Bungay Black Dog Runners, and has the feel of small, intimate race.

I wish I'd had more time to explore Bungay which sits on the River Waveney and has a fascinating history. A weekly Thursday market has been held since 1382 on the site of the Butter Cross which was rebuilt following the Great Fire of Bungay in 1688. St Mary's Church dominates the local landscape and dates from the 12th Century. But above all, Bungay is famous for a visit by Black Shuck, the "Black Dog of Bungay" in 1577 who, during a violent storm, ran around the church and terrified the congregation. The legend has continued to fascinate generations of townsfolk ever since.

Fortunately, there were no black dogs to nip at runners' ankles on the day of the race. But it was a nippy morning for running. Almost 600 runners took part in the race which was staged on a fast countryside course, with a few testing hills along tight, windy lanes.

After a rubbish training session three nights earlier when I ran tired like a sack of potatoes, I surprised myself with 102nd place in 1 hour 28 minutes, which was pretty respectable running in the circumstances. Had I run a little quicker I would have picked up a spot prize which the guy ahead of me won – a box of racing gels to keep up energy levels during a race.

Suffolk is so pretty at this time of year. Snowdrops decorated the fields, and rolling countryside dotted with distinctive Norman churches, plus the occasional windmill. The night before the race, Liz and I stayed in a 400-year-old house in Pulham Market which used to be the village bakery. It is a beautiful home. The Old Bakery was established in 1580, in the reign of Queen Elizabeth I, to become the main bakery for the area. It was in continuous use for over 400 years. The last baker retired in 1951.

The house itself is a listed building, constructed of an oak timber frame with walls of wattle and daub, and we stayed in a lovely little room at the far end of the house. One of the owners, Martin, is a former master chef, so when he asked for our breakfast order on the morning of the race, I said porridge. Come Sunday morning, he had slaved for hours over a traditional porridge cooked with salt. Yuk! I must make a mental note to myself; avoid at all costs salted porridge before a race. No make that; avoid at all costs salted porridge...ever!

10. The Terminator @ Pewsey, Wiltshire.

A WEEK later for the last week in February, I found myself on all fours, climbing a fiendish hill in the middle of the Wiltshire countryside, cursing myself for ever having entered the race.

I was fatigued, my legs and shoes were caked in mud, and the insides of my knees were smarting with cuts – the result of an unfortunate fall a few miles back. Meanwhile, standing at the top of the hill, cheerfully waving at me like a boy scout who's found the escape route was my mate Ian Witcher. "C'mon Dave, hurry up. I've found someone to take our photograph," he shouted. "It will make a great shot for the paper."

I crawled my way to the summit, tried to raise a smile for the guy with the box brownie and before I knew it Ian, the fastest postman on the south coast, was off like, well, like a postman being chased by a rabid dog!

This was The Terminator, a fearsome 11-and-a-half mile cross country race based in Pewsey near Marlborough. It is a race which takes no prisoners and is a real test of stamina and endurance; both physical and mental.

Ian, an all-round good guy but pretty quick when he gets going, had agreed to run the course with me. "Go easy, don't go off too quick," was his advice to me and fellow Southampton Running Club member, Rob Parkinson, a detective constable with Hampshire Police.

A year ago when Ian ran the Terminator, it was so cold that even the brass monkeys stayed indoors. At least if we had got those conditions this time around it would have made the ground firmer. Within the first mile we had run through a mini quagmire by a ditch and picked our way along a mud-strewn path by the Kennet and Avon canal which was like a chocolate skating rink. It was a wonder no-one slipped and fell into the drink.

This was only an appetiser for worst things to come because at three miles some wise guy had stuck up a sign saying "that was only a warm up". We then entered a narrow and slippery path called the Gully. All you could do was to run straight through the mud, there was little point trying to avoid it. But even that had its hazards. In some places, the mud was so thick you could feel it pulling your shoes off. It was thick and gloopy, resisting every attempt to lift your foot and press forward. Then, as I tried to pick my way through one tricky part, I unceremoniously slipped and fell flat on my back. It hurt, but there was no time to stop. You had to pick yourself up and drag yourself up the slimy slope.

Avoiding the mud was impossible, navigating your way around those exhausted runners floundering in the stuff was even more difficult. At every turn there was a challenge. The Coomb, Dodge Sh**ty and the Terminator Hill itself. At least on the higher ground there was no mud, but the climbs were tough and back-breaking. For the rapid descents it was a question of keeping your balance and picking the right path as your top half tried to overtake your legs. The slow progress uphill meant there was plenty of time for banter with runners who struggled beside you. We were in this together, encouraging each other, and stopping to help those who fell.

The Terminator was an unadulterated test of survival. With ten miles on the clock, the end was apparently in sight, and that's when the Sting in the Tail bit you firmly on the bum. Right next door to the famous White Horse carved in the Wiltshire countryside was another on-all-fours climb. You ran down this gentle ridge believing you were heading back to Pewsey when around the corner you were greeted by this morale-sapping torture.

It was a run of attrition, a battle to get to the top and down. But I made it, heaven knows how. Finally, I was on the way home, but not before visiting the infamous Shoe Wash which consisted of jumping into the waist-high freezing waters of the River Avon; three steps in and out.

Ian and Rob had finished a few of minutes ahead of me as I plodded home in 1 hour 52 minutes. Both guys were there at the end, looking sickeningly fresh as if they'd been out for a morning stroll. "Enjoy that one?" asked Ian cheerily. "Yes," I replied.

Though The Terminator was hard, the sense of achievement at finishing was enormous. Taking home the t-shirt afforded a wonderful feeling of immense satisfaction from this race of character. Above all, I was two months into the project, 10 races down, and 70 to go!

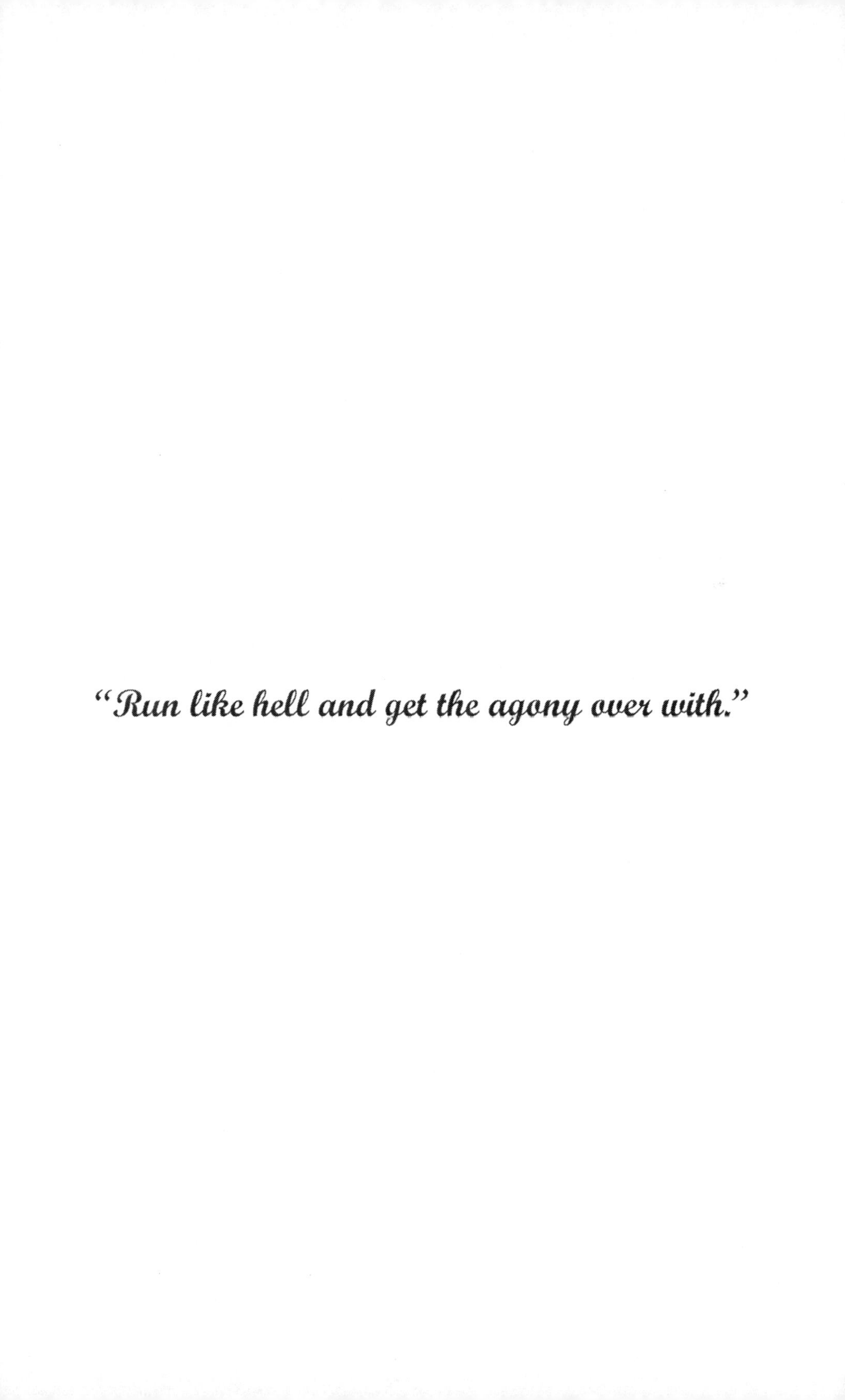

"Run like hell and get the agony over with."

MAR2007

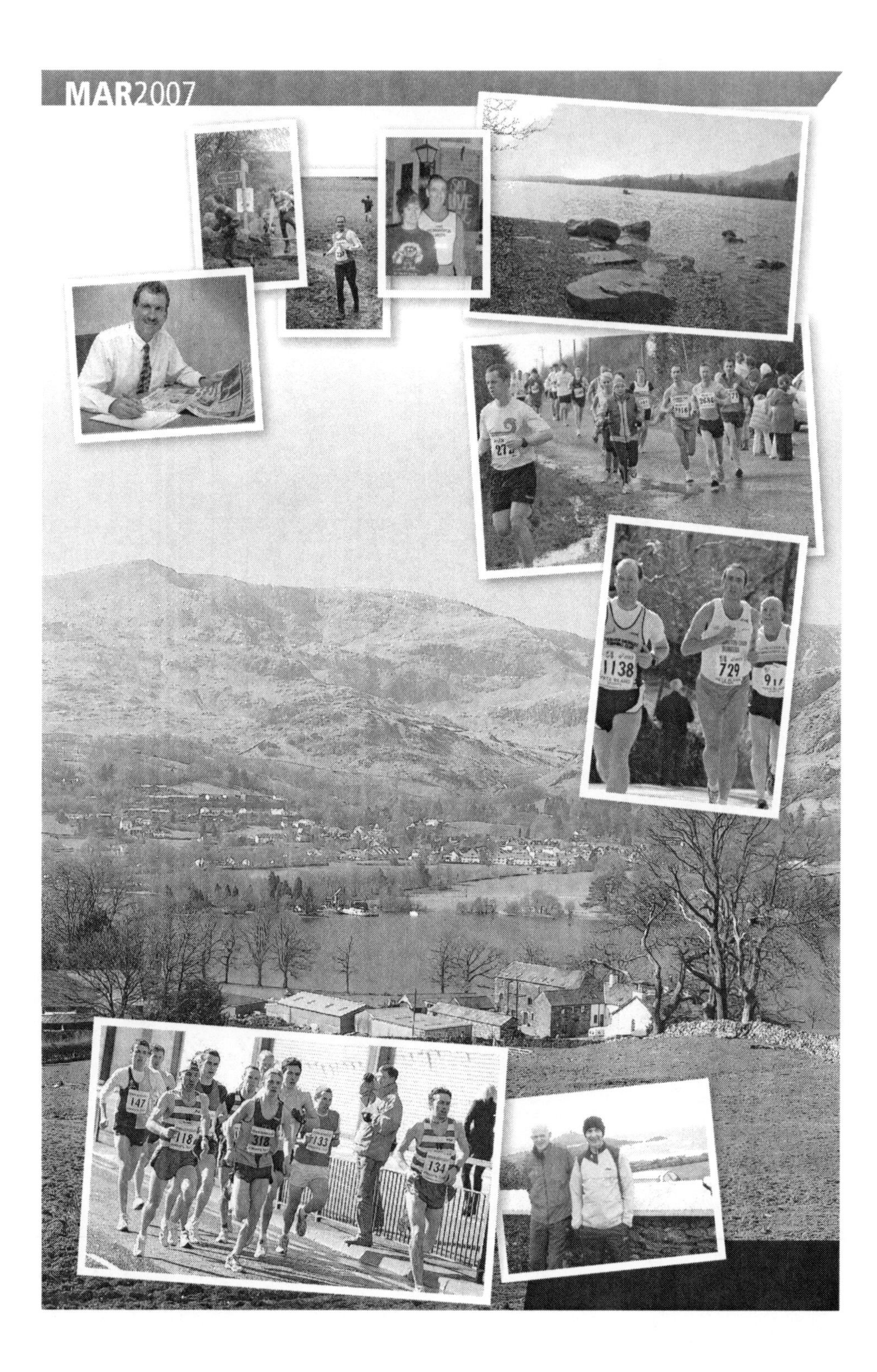

MARCH

11. Vectis Lunatics' Full Moon Run @ Ryde, Isle of Wight.

VARIETY is the proverbial spice of life, and among the many ingredients to this year-long running challenge was the need to experience different types of racing; road, fell, cross country and hashing.

Now I had first heard about the sport of hashing during a two-year stint working abroad in the Persian Gulf. There I met a couple of guys who were members of the Bahrain Hash House Harriers. I had never been to a hash before – the word conjures up sordid images of all sorts of illegal activities, usually taking place in some 1960s' free-love bar in Amsterdam – and so, purely for the readers' interest and my own education, I was determined during this mad-cap year not to miss out on this journey of running exploration.

For millions of runners around the world, hashing is very much part of their life. Unkindly described by some as "the drinking club with a running problem", the Hash House Harriers is essentially a social club with a running element so, perhaps, the deep-rooted morals should be "Running with Attitude" or "You Have to Earn Your Drink"! The Hash has its humble beginnings in what is now Malaysia thanks to an Englishman whose parents clearly had a cruel touch when it came to handing out middle names for their children - Albert Stephen Ignatius Gispert.

Runs involving groups of unfit expatriates following a paper trail were a pretty common pastime in colonial Malaya back in the 1930s. But hashing got its name from a place called the Selangor Club Chambers which, due to its unimaginative and monotonous food, was commonly referred to by the British expats as the "Hash House".

Having a fondness for the paper chase, Gispert, who was later killed in the fighting in Singapore in 1942, gathered together a group of expats - including Cecil Lee, 'Horse' Thomson and 'Torch' Bennett - to form a running group in Kuala Lumpur that would later leave a worldwide legacy.

There are numerous tales which have been doctored and embellished about the origins of hashing, but my favourite is the one that fed up by the food and the lack of exercise, the fellowship decided to go out for a run. They rummaged through the kitchens of the Selangor Club, found some flour before one of their number began laying a trail through the countryside for the others to follow, adding false leads and loopbacks just for the hell of it. As so often happens, good intentions can lead to an evil end, and these social runs would invariably climax with plenty of wining and dining to celebrate what was very much a social occasion.

Today, that philosophy continues the world over with hundreds of thousands of hashing clubs. So one bitterly cold Thursday evening in March, I caught the ferry from Southampton across the Solent to the Isle of Wight to catch up with members of the Vectis Lunatics Hash House Harriers for their monthly Full Moon Hash.

When we met outside a pub in Ryde, there were about 40 runners all raring to go for the 7pm start. It didn't help that my two hosts, Richard Pearson - hash name P-Rick - and his girlfriend Deanna Westwood - hash name Bumps - arrived late at the pub, with myself in tow, having picked me up from the ferry terminal at East Cowes.

Richard, a 51-year-old greeting card salesman, really got it in the neck from his mates for being late. A pretty decent runner who has posted a 3 hour 30 minute marathon time, Richard had earlier that afternoon set the evening's course. So while he was parking the car, Deanna and myself, armed with torches, set off in pursuit of the rest of the bunch who went shooting off around the dark streets of Ryde.

For me it was a case of picking up the rules as we went along. Hashing involves following a trail which has been laid by flour. On street corners, by lamp posts, in the middle of paths, you would spot tiny blobs of flour, and various flour-drawn symbols. When a trail was found, cries of "on on" could be heard. Heaven knows what the locals thought of these antics as they headed for their evening outing to the bingo!

False trails were occasionally marked as hashers found themselves running up blind alleys to be greeted by a flour bar. Fishhooks would be laid, forcing the faster runners to turn round and rejoin the back of the group. It was a classic paper trail, but made with flour.

The Vectis Lunatics are part of the Isle of Wight Hash House Harriers who run regularly each Sunday for up to two hours. It is a gathering not only for runners since there are walkers too. The once a month Full Moon Hash is more a runner's hash which lasts an hour, tending to cover a course of between three to four miles.

Richard had chosen a nasty little route. I had brought road shoes thinking we would be trailing round streets, little expecting we would be running across muddy, dark fields. We clocked up 3.5 miles, finishing back at the pub for "down downs". "Hashing is not a sport, it is an attitude," Richard explained later, as I was being chatted up by a hideous young thing in the pub. Hideous Young Thing was wondering what I was doing scribbling away in a notebook. With a tongue stud, wild hair, and perfume which could paralyse a bull from 50 yards, she was the date from hell. Richard smiled as he revelled in my discomfort, but would do nothing to bail me out and just continued the conversation as HYT swooned in the corner. I could swear she was teasing me with the tongue stud!

"Some people get it, others don't," he continued, as the HYT wild child started getting too close for comfort, her Eau de Sewer was becoming overpowering. "It's not competitive, hashing is a social run. I work all week and the last thing I want to do on a Sunday, or on a Full Moon Hash, is to be competitive. Running ability is not important. You have to be able to laugh at yourself and with others, and also have fun. We have runners who come along to join us but who simply don't get it. They come along once then we don't see them again. You need a sense of humour. We're all good friends; there is a tremendous amount of camaraderie."

That camaraderie overflowed in the pub afterwards with drinks and food laid on by the landlady. I managed to get out of the dangerous date with HYT by telling her I was gay and impotent! Meanwhile the Master of Ceremonies for the evening, who went by the Hash name of 'Shergar', picked out various sinners to down glasses of different liquids. Richard was named and shamed for his lateness. I was involved in a lemonade drinking race with a fellow hasher called Betty. Our crimes? Being teetotal!

The evening was great fun, this was what running is all about. One of the reasons I undertook the project was to reinvigorate my running. My sport had become too obsessed with personal bests, forever looking at the watch and constantly checking my race position. Instead, here was a group of people, mostly middle aged, but with a sprinkling of young 'uns and crinklies, who enjoy their sport for the hell of it. Yes, competition is the lifeblood of sport, but there is also an important place for the likes of hashing and the good guys and gals at the Vectis Lunatics.

12. Ballycotton 10 @ Ballycotton, County Cork, Republic of Ireland

OPENING the lightweight curtains at Mrs Leahy's bed and breakfast with the wind rattling against the wooden frames, the omens were not looking good. All night long, driving rain had been lashing against the window panes and the creaking wooden panels of the isolated 18th century Georgian guest house which sat proudly on a hill overlooking Ballycotton Bay. Wiping away the condensation to peer through the gap, it was hard to pick out the white-bricked lighthouse, its red beacon shrouded in the storm which was raging from the Atlantic Ocean.

Welcome to the Emerald Isle and County Cork early on a Sunday morning in March with the sweet smell of bacon and sausages wafting upstairs. Had this been a holiday, then a warm bed and a few extra hours' kip would have been a more attractive proposition. But this was my first trip to Ireland, here to take part in the Ballycotton 10 which was this year celebrating its 30th anniversary.

It was an August evening back in 1977 when in Ballycotton the first-ever organised road race in modern times took place. A five mile blitzkrieg, it was won by Ray Treacy, brother of John, the Irish Olympic Marathon silver medallist from Los Angeles in 1984 and a two-time winner of the World Cross Country title.

The following March, 31 runners, all men, took part in a ten-mile race in Ballycotton and by 1993 the race had grown when 1,000 runners raced for the first time. Since then, with the advent of the running boom in Ireland, and despite virtually no advertising, numbers taking part have grown to over 2,800 finishers in 2006.

The Irish running legend Sonia O'Sullivan who hails from the nearby town of Cobh won the prestigious race back in 2001, and for the 21st anniversary celebrations in 1998, the President of Ireland, Mary McAleese, attended to watch husband Martin complete the ten miles in a respectable time. Now the almost impossible task facing the organisers is to devise a system that will limit the number of entrants to a manageable level, while keeping most people happy!

Its success is down to one man, the untiring and indefatigable race director John Walshe who, even on that miserable morning, had been out at 6am in the bleak weather checking the entire route of the course.

What strikes you as bizarre is why hold a race at all in an out-of-the-way Irish village? Okay, so there's 500 euros up for grabs for the first man and woman, and a souvenir mug for us mortals, but John reckoned the success was down to Ballycotton's unique, friendly atmosphere. It's a 10-mile party which runs across the weekend with many visitors vowing to return again.

On our first evening in Ballycotton, Liz and I had taken a run-in to the village which lies at the end of a peninsula. There really is nothing to the place. Blink and you'll miss it. There's one hotel, a school, a couple of shops, plus a few bars lining a main street which rolls into and out of the village. Homes nestle snuggly into the hillside sat above a small harbour which provides sanctuary to half a dozen fishing vessels. How was Ballycotton possibly going to cope with more than 2,000 runners from across Ireland, plus a couple of hundred enthusiasts who had ventured over the Irish Sea?

In a small bar, we caught up with a lovely man called Jim McMurtry, a friend of John's. Liz and I were the only out-of-towners, but Jim, a tall, thin and wiry man, with a softly-spoken Irish accent was warm and welcoming. "What yer having?" he asked. "I'm on the Lucozade, always do before a race." It was hard to believe any Irish pub would be stocking bottles of Lucozade, let alone find an Irishman who preferred the fizzy orange stuff to the sacred black nectar. Jim had spent 20 years living in Southampton, so when he had heard a few months back that we were flying over from the south coast, the Saints-supporting Irishman was keen to meet up. "I used to work in Southampton and I've still got family there. You name a civic building in Southampton, and I probably fitted the windows," he boasted. Jim reminded me that his friend John Walshe also had Southampton connections since one of his uncles was a Catholic priest based in the city until his retirement in the 1990s.

It was a beautiful Spring evening as we walked back to our car to return to the B&B. County Cork had been bathed in brilliant March sunshine when Liz and I visited the delightful town of Cobh and the Queenstown Story museum. This building told the story of how three million folk emigrated from the port, many to America, particularly between the great famine of 1848 to 1850.

On our way out of the bar, Jim warned us how bad the weather would be for race day. "Wrap up warm," was his worldly wise parting shot. And true to his word, less than 12 hours later I was taking in the bleak rain-sodden view from the bedroom window as a brutal south-east gale whipped off the sea, while the comforting smell of a traditional Irish cooked breakfast drifted upstairs from Mrs Leahy's kitchen. The locals told me later that this was the worst race day weather since 1989, the year of the "Big Wind".

The one consolation was that the race start wasn't until 1.30pm which meant there was no excuse not to take in some of the Emerald Isle hospitality. It wouldn't have been decent to do otherwise, would it? First there was a classic oatmeal porridge, following by a full Irish breakfast, and don't spare the trimmings. Chatting to some of the other 'B&B'ers, I managed over breakfast to become an honorary member of the Irish Osteoporosis Society, rewarded with a prized car parking pass. Parking places are scant on the Ballycotton peninsular, so buses ferried runners into Ballycotton from a plethora of car parks dotted along the coastline. Thanks to my new exalted position earned less than 24 hours after arriving in Ireland and armed with a prized parking permit, this enabled me to bypass the Garda roadblocks set up on the edge of the village. Despite these hard-earned privileges, parking in Ballycotton was problematic. However, just as I was despairing of finding the smallest of spaces, close to the harbour wall we spotted our pal Jim who ushered us to a parking place close to his. I protested about parking on a double yellow line.

"Oh, be gone wid yer," said Jim. "This is Ireland for heaven's sake. We don't take notice of silly things like yellow lines."

Though the rain had relented, the clouds remained a threatening grey as a fair old wind whipped off the headland. Very soon, Ballycotton began filling up with track-suited runners. Television crews were there, so were radio reporters and newspaper photographers. The queues for the loos in the village school snaked round the hopscotch markings in the playground. Because of flooding in fields on the outskirts of Ballycotton where the park and ride was set up, some runners had been held up, so the start was delayed by a quarter of an hour. No-one was fussed. The atmosphere was relaxed as a regular stream of announcements were relayed over the Tannoy.

Come race time, classical Irish music played loudly over the speakers – yards down the road Freddie Mercury was belting out "Don't Stop Me Now" over another rig. There was a smile on the face of every runner packed into Ballycotton's main street just as the sun appeared for the first time.

The first mile was downhill and I had been warned to go easy. The entire ten-mile race route was sealed off from traffic so the narrow country lanes were lined with enthusiastic and vocal spectators. What was jaw-dropping was the standard of running. The first 65 runners finished in under an hour, which is lightning quick and my time of 71 minutes was well off the pace. I ran with a bright young thing called Loretto Duggan from St Mary's AC; blonde and beautiful and with a Christian name which sounded like an Italian ice cream. She was strong too. Despite trying to out-do and lose each other on the course, we entered the final hill into Ballycotton stride by stride. Gallantly, I sprinted past the Bambi-legged youngster to win by a measly second.

John Walshe and his team put on a first-class race. It is well organised, great course, friendly atmosphere, superb competition which sticks firmly to the race motto – a classic race at a classic distance.

13. Banbury 15 @ Banbury, Oxfordshire.

PAUL Bithell was a wonderful man, my only regret was that I never got to know him better. He was a fantastic journalist who I worked with in Portsmouth in the early 1990s and who possessed a wonderful temperament. The only time the Welsh wizard got riled was on the football field where, as a central defender, he simply didn't have a clue how to play the offside trap.

Paul later moved to Oxfordshire to become editor of the Banbury Guardian, and in 1999, while training for a triathlon, he was diagnosed with a brain tumour. Paul was a fighter, and he fought an astonishing battle. Driven by journalistic instinct, he was compelled to write about what subsequently happened to him; what he called the rollercoaster ride of experiences following that fateful day. During chemotheraphy, he maintained his good humour, dignity and courage throughout. An enthusiastic charity worker, he became the driving force behind a newspaper campaign to complete the last leg of an £80,000 appeal to fund a new Macmillan nurse for the Banbury area. At one stage, we thought Paul was going to beat the big C. In his final article, Paul described how lucky he felt he had been as an early prognosis had given him just three months to live. Three years had passed but on Christmas Eve in 2002, Paul died aged 44. Fast forward to 2007, and that week I had also celebrated my 44th birthday. The age comparisons provided a sobering thought which was the wake-up call I needed at a time when three months and just 12 races into the 80-race challenge, I was feeling a little listless and lethargic.

I was in Banbury where each year they hold a two-mile fun run around the town's park in memory of Paul. I had been expecting to run a notorious race in Devon called The Grizzly, but this gruelling 20-miler along windswept cliffs and down muddy dales had been postponed with one of the strangest excuses ever offered – because of a beached cargo ship. The route of The Grizzly takes in Branscombe Beach which in March was still strewn with battered metal containers from the 62,000-tonne MSC Napoli that had in January been holed in storms in the English Channel. It was here that television cameras from around the world descended on the beach to capture images of wide-eyed scavengers running off with all sorts of goods from the containers including BMW motorbikes, wine, face cream and nappies. Police were looking out for an incontinent, drunken biker with a nice complexion!

So instead of venturing to South Devon, I had chosen instead to race in Banbury on a gorgeous sunny day for running. The two-mile fun run would have been nice, but I chose to test myself over the longer 15-mile distance. It felt like the first day of Spring which brought out a few strange-looking runners – one was sporting an iPod with the headphone wire taped to his cheek, and another looked like Dennis the Menace wearing knee-length shorts, a buttoned shirt and a back to front cap.

The route took us out of Banbury, north across the M40 motorway and along winding country lanes. It was a hard race with two pretty stiff hills thrown in. Early on I tagged along with a local fireman called Rob. We were targeting another strangely attired runner, this one was wearing a thick t-shirt and tracksuit bottoms on a sweltering hot day. "That lad's taking the mick," moaned Rob, dressed in a t-shirt and shorts, as we pushed our way up one sharp hill. "We're running at a pretty good pace, sweating buckets and look at him. I'm not having that." And with that Rob was off in pursuit eventually managing to overtake tracksuit man.

I passed the guy a few miles later before settling into the race in with a lady called Pat, a mother-of-three from High Wycombe, who was also training for the London Marathon. We talked about her family and work, how she managed to juggle those commitments with her running, and how she was looking forward to the big race. Amazingly, the miles rattled by, the couple of big climbs were easily overcome, and towards the end of the run we were catching and passing runners pretty comfortably.

At the finish on the walk back to the car park, chomping away on a big block of Toblerone which had been dished out at the end of the race, I thought about Paul, his ready smile and wit. He would have enjoyed that race, he would have revelled in the enormous challenge which I was facing and determined to conquer.

14. Glenariff Mountain Race @ Waterfoot, Northern Ireland.

TWO weeks after running around the Republic of Ireland, I was back in the Emerald Isle, this time north of the border in Ulster – where else could you choose to be over the St Patrick's Weekend?

Thanks to my generous sponsors Flybe, who were providing all flights to me out of England, I flew into the nattily named George Best Belfast City Airport on Friday evening straight from work, got an upgrade on my hire car, and then set out on the M2 motorway north to Ballymena skirting the bright lights of the capital. I was due to meet my host for the weekend, Mark Alexander, organiser of the first of two weekend races, who had insisted that I stay with his family when he learned of my trip to Northern Ireland.

Driving past the impressive Odyssey Arena, lit up on Belfast's waterfront, I had a horrible feeling in the pit of my stomach. It brought back wretched memories of school French exchanges when for a fortnight you would be thrown with a family you had never met before, who you might not get on with and in a country where you didn't understand the language too well – all broad similarities with my plight in Northern Ireland!

Mark and I met in a dark and deserted car park just as the local KFC was clearing out. We drove in convoy to Mark's smart home on the outskirts of Ballymena where wife Valerie and their young children Katie and Emily had just arrived home fresh from attending a Brownies' awards evening. Any anxieties I had nurtured about this "blind date" were quickly extinguished over coffee in the kitchen where Mark and Valerie were wonderfully genial hosts serving up good conversation and Barm Brack; a traditional Irish bread, a sort of fruit loaf.

As a child of the 70s, the troubles in Northern Ireland dominated the consciousness. Grainy, black and white television pictures of the British Army with riot shields being showered by stone throwers. News programmes dominated by bombings both in Ulster and on the mainland, hearing the harsh oratory of Ian Paisley and seeing the images of the balaclava-wearing IRA volunteers brandishing fearsome-looking Kalashnikov rifles.

That St Patrick's weekend, elections to the Northern Ireland assembly had just taken place yet it was still disquieting to see the smiling face of Sinn Fein president Gerry Adams staring at you from a poster asking for your vote. Take a drive down Belfast's Falls Road and you're thrown into a timewarp of troubles not long since past.

The Falls Road – its Irish name Bóthar na bhFál means road of the hedgerows – is synonymous with the worst violence during the troubles in Northern Ireland. During my weekend in the province, I took a drive down what was once a staunch Republican stronghold to see for myself what it was about. Even today, the Republican roots remain strong. Reminders of the troubles are clear to see. Black flags, another legacy to those dark days, still hang from some homes.

"Twenty-five years of resistance, 25 years more if need-be" cried one of the murals which lined this part of West Belfast. The yellow Harland & Wolff cranes dominate the skyline, yet you could see in the capital and elsewhere in the province how Northern Ireland is trying hard to shed the old clothes of the past to build a new and vibrant place.

The ugly redbrick buildings and Coronation Street-style home remain in some parts, but these are fast being replaced by modern glass buildings, office complexes and shopping malls. Wherever I went, there was a renewed sense of optimism. All the false dawns had been replaced with a genuine belief that peace could rein as Protestants and Catholics lived alongside each other.

Back in Ballymena, I tagged along with Mark and Valerie to a St Patrick's Day party where I bumped into a policeman who served with the Royal Ulster Constabulary during the troubles. He was cautious about saying too much. I wanted to know what it had been like then, for him to reflect on the enormous pressure which he and his family had faced as a serving member of the RUC. "We still get our fair share of trouble," he said, as we went up for seconds on the dessert table. "But at least you are no longer getting up in the morning and checking under your car in case someone's put a bomb there. That prospect keeps you alert and awake first thing in the morning."

After a good night's sleep in Ballymena, I joined Mark on the Saturday morning for a 15-mile drive to the town of Waterfoot which lies on the north-eastern coast. In the distance across the North Channel, the narrow strait linking the Irish Sea with the North Atlantic Ocean, you could just pick out the headland of the Mull of Kintyre on Scotland's western coastline, some 13 miles distant. This side of the water, the mountain of Glenariff, one of the nine glens of Antrim standing at over 1,000 feet tall, dominated the spectacular skyline. This was a most beautiful and tranquil place.

Sadly the weather did not match the beauty as, during the morning, stormy weather closed in. I helped Mark and some of his clubmates from Ballymena Runners to help get the race ready at St Patrick's Primary School. At 1pm, 70 runners lined up for the start. Although the rain had held off, the winds were gusting.

We set off along the Ulster Way, a flat two-mile cross country route to the foot of Glenariff. From there, it was a mile-long climb to the summit. It was hard, it was cruel, it was back-breaking. You could barely run up some parts of the climb and at times we were on all-fours trying to pick out a route. Finally I made it to the top of the climb which was the easy part. Now came the descent which bordered on the suicidal.

At the time of the race I was reading Richard Askwith's acclaimed sports book, "Feet In The Clouds" which centres on fell running. It's an acclaimed piece of literature which I felt was tedious, tending to regard the achievements of any runner who does not run the fells as unworthy. What Askwith's book does describe supremely well is the history of the sport, picking out the courage of fell runners who throw themselves off mountainsides at breakneck speeds, where injury is regarded an occupational hazard and speed the absolute key. To them and those experienced fell runners who hared past me, I give my utmost respect. Their bravery and balance was supreme, their downhill speed simply gobsmacking.

The rocks and grassland was soaking wet. Several times I painfully went over on my backside, slipping and sliding down the mountain. Rocks were strewn everywhere as I galloped downhill out of control. I passed one lady who was gingerly making her way down. She explained that she was saving herself for the London Marathon in six weeks' time. "Me too," I shouted. "Jesus," she cried back. "So I'm not the only ejit on this bloody mountain breaking my neck training for a marathon!"

Fortunately, the only injuries were pride through the frequent falls on the 5.92 mile run where I finished a poor 51st out of 71 runners. Uniquely, the prize for every finisher was a sack of potatoes from the local sponsors and the post-race spread of sandwiches, cake and tea was absolutely magnificent. Ballymena Runners also presented me with a generous cheque to the National Autistic Society in Northern Ireland, which I was delighted to receive on their behalf.

15, Jimmy's 10 @ Downpatrick, Northern Ireland.

THE morning after St Patrick's Day, I was up early for the hour-long drive to Downpatrick which lies in the south-eastern corner of the province in County Antrim. This was the venue for Jimmy's 10, a 10km race which began in 1999 as a memorial to Jimmy Murray, a popular man in East Down who was greatly involved with developing athletes, particularly young athletes, in the province. Jimmy, who was a teacher at St Columba's College in Portaferry, was the driving force behind the founding of East Down Athletic Club in 1987. He died from cancer in July 1998 at the age of 49 within three months of diagnosis and so the race remembers his work.

On this Northern Ireland leg of the trip I met so many lovely characters. One was Joe Quinn, the race organiser, who was surrounded by his posse of gorgeous daughters. He had also taken a close interest in my project, and somehow had got my story and grinning photograph plastered across the back page of the local newspaper, the Down Democrat.

He had also handed me race number 1 which was a bit of a millstone around my neck. With my sharp Stubbington Green vest which none of the locals recognised and flashy Asics kit, you could see the race whippets eyeing me up wondering how fast was the new competition. On the start line overlooking St Patrick's Cathedral I decided to play the game. Ten minutes before the start I stood on the front of the start line, and then jogged ahead into the open road to go through the motions of a rigorous warm-up and strides. You could feel the harsh glares from the fast runners, and sense their sneaked conversations. Who is this interloper? How fast do you think he runs the 10km? Is he an international? Just then, the starter called us to the start line and I walked back slowly with great concentration, stretching and flexing my neck muscles and chewing gum as I strode towards the throng . The guys right on the front row courteously opened up a gap on the front line for me to line up next to them, but I just said "excuse me" and kept on walking to take my rightful place near the back of the field. That had them worried!

As for the race itself, there was a nasty surprise early on with a shocking hill climb to the cathedral, before the race headed out to the River Quoile and along a windy path by the nature reserve. It was a very pleasant run around Downpatrick finishing along the main street. Joe gave me a bag full of goodies to take home and later presented me with a cheque for the Hampshire Autistic Society. Say what you like about the Irish, but they do put on a good feast after the race. More tea, cake and sandwiches; it was an impressive spread.

Reminiscences of a troubled past flooded back while I was in Downpatrick. How much has peace moved on? How much tolerance and understanding had there been? After all, the race route passed close to Ballydougan Road where, in 1990, four Ulster Defence Regiment soldiers were killed by a 1,000lb IRA landmine. "It's why some people here find it so hard to move on," one local told me, having admitted, somewhat remarkably, that he had been in the Ulster Defence Regiment. "Where you ran today by the River Quoile there is a telephone box and it was there that two policemen were shot during the troubles. It is right that we move on. Thank God we live in peace, but while you try very hard to forgive, you can never forget."

Later on as I was tucking into a plateful of sandwiches in the sports hall, another lady, whose young son had recently been diagnosed with autism, came up to me with her husband. She was beside herself with worry. She explained how they were finding it difficult to cope with the prospect of their son's autism, not knowing what to do or who to turn to. "It has changed our lives," she said. "I'm not sure what I am going to do. I can't sleep, I'm always worrying. Our son so depends on us. We look after him all the time and the thing which worries me most is who is going to look after him when I am no longer on this earth. It breaks my heart. It makes me cry."

We spoke for a while. I tried to reassure the couple with my own experiences of my son Ross – telling them of the hammer blow I felt learning my child had autism, how this changed your life forever; but that life is always tinged with hope and very soon you build in coping mechanisms. "You mustn't look too far ahead because you don't know how your son's autism will manifest itself in future years," I said. "Many are able to lead independent lives, some will adapt. Where there's life, there's hope." And with that, the couple wrote out a cheque for the Hampshire Autistic Society, put it in my palm, shook my hand and walked away hand in hand.

It was a quite amazing weekend, a wonderful place, outstanding scenery and a time when I met some truly memorable people.

As I walked back to my car for the trip to Belfast, I spotted a poster on a wall at the leisure centre. It made me think of that lady and her autistic child, it made me think of my situation with Ross, and I reflected on how the face of Northern Ireland has changed so markedly over the past decade with these words: "Within me is infinite power, before me is endless possibility, around me is boundless opportunity. So, why should I fear?"

16. Coniston 14 @ Coniston, Cumbria.

ONE of the biggest challenges of the project was juggling work with the travelling, running and sheer organisation. My job as a journalist was demanding enough without adding anything extra into the mix. At times it was exhausting and just before the last weekend in March I was working in Poole running examinations for journalists. At the end of a long Friday on the south coast, I dashed out of the building armed with a bundle of papers to begin a tiring six-hour car journey to the Lake District for a race the following morning.

Grabbing an overpriced sausage roll, a packet of crisps and some tart-tasting orange juice from one of those overpriced motorway service stations,

I began the long drive. Earlier in the day Liz had almost been forced to remortgage the house in order to buy a train ticket from the south coast to Cumbria. Shortly before midnight, she was just about to go to bed when I finally arrived at the B&B on the edge of Lake Coniston. The prospect loomed of another challenging race, the Coniston 14 – but that was another day.

Saturday dawned and it was a beauty. It was unusual to be racing at 11am on a Saturday morning, since most of my races during the year were scheduled for the Sunday. But what the heck?! This was springtime in a mini paradise with temperatures touching the late 50s Fahrenheit. I wondered whether there could be a more scenic or picturesque race in the British Isles? For runners feeling depressed and despondent about their sport, lacking motivation to run, or maybe bored with the same old diet of predictable races, then Coniston offers the perfect antidote. If life in general is getting you into a rut, then this would be where your doctor would prescribe you to get away from it all; clean air, spectacular views and a wonderful atmosphere. This was one the most uplifting races I have run. The most satisfying, definitely the most scenic, in fact, probably my best race ever.

It helped that this delightful Cumbrian town was bathed in gorgeous March sunshine. Tufts of snow settled near the 2,635 foot peak of the imperious Old Man of Coniston, dominating a skyline of craggy peaks which formed an impressive bowl around the lake where a few boats, tethered to orange buoys, swayed in the slight breeze. Coniston Water, forever etched in British history as the place where speed enthusiast Donald Campbell was killed in 1967 attempted to improve his world water speed record in Bluebird, was looking serene. The lake was also to be our marker on this 14-mile race, well 13.8-miles to be precise, around the country lanes which forms its boundary.

The Coniston 14, which has been running for 25 years raising over £100,000 for local charities, is a testing hilly run. None of the hills are particularly cruel, though they would be if the race was run clockwise around Coniston Water. Instead, these are short, sharp, challenging rises, which are balanced by gentle downhills.

Stone walls lined the race route which started in Coniston and headed towards the village of Torver. It was congested at the start along the tight and windy narrow lanes, but soon the race field spread out. To our left was the sight of the lake, to the right were the rocky mountains; the sun shone, the breeze made sure it wasn't too hot; this was perfect running weather.

The race attracts runners from all over the country and no wonder; even the landlady where I was staying took part. There is a strong tradition of fell running in these parts where men are men who eat up the steep climbs and think nothing of throwing themselves down the most ferocious of slopes.

The build on some of the runners with their powerful thighs, strong upper body and occasional tattoo was impressive – and those were only the women! These were runners to be reckoned with. The first 49 finishers were under 90 minutes. It is a debatable point, but is the standard of running stronger in the north than it is in the south?

The Coniston 14 has been going since 1982 and it is very much a race staged by the collective goodwill of the village. The organisers had been forced to make some late changes following the sudden death of David Clarke. David was a man well known in these parts; a race organiser of events such as the Chernobyl 10km near Preston, the Caldervale 10 and the Garstang 10km, a course measurer and a reliable producer of race results. He was one of a band of no-nonsense volunteers who turned up to races whatever the weather to get the event on.

Just three days before the Coniston 14, David, who was 53, fell through his garage roof which he was repairing and sustained a massive head injury. He was rushed to the Royal Preston Hospital for an emergency operation, but died in the early hours of Saturday morning just hours before the race.

Brian Porter, organiser of the nearby Freckleton Half Marathon, was a close friend of David's: "I received a telephone call from David's wife, Dianne, at 6.40am that morning and she asked me to let some people know. These people were stepping in to do the results at Coniston 14. I had no plans to go to Coniston but it just seemed to be the right place to be that day.

"David did many things on the spur of the moment so I guess it was fitting really that our decision to give him one minute's applause on the start line was also a spur of the moment decision made by myself and Ron McAndrew."

Brian read an address at David's funeral a few weeks later, speaking stirringly about a man who he first got to know as "the bloke in the corner doing the results". "David was the man who recorded forever just how slowly I had run," he told the congregation. "He produced results magnificently. You could rely on them being on his web site within hours of a race finishing. And he could do so much with those results. If you wanted to wind up your mate he would happily change a name, an age, even a person's gender for a laugh. Sometimes though, he'd 'forget' to change the details back and the poor unfortunate would appear on the results like that for months! And whenever David was at a race, Dianne wasn't far away. Often she was timekeeping and keeping us in order at the finish, while knitting a jumper. Oh yes, this was a double act and what a double act it was!

"'Leave it with me and I'll sort it' is a fitting epitaph. As a course measurer he was second to none. One phone call was all it took and he'd be out there in all weathers to make sure the organiser had an accurate distance. Any doubts over the accuracy of a course distance were quickly dispelled with the words 'Dave Clarke measured that'."

The sun shone that day for Dave Clarke on what was a glorious run around the lake, and I was sad the race came to an end as we wound our way back into the delightful town of Coniston for the final stretch home. This was one race which would rank as my favourite of the entire running year.

"It hurts up to a point and then it doesn't get any worse."

APR2007

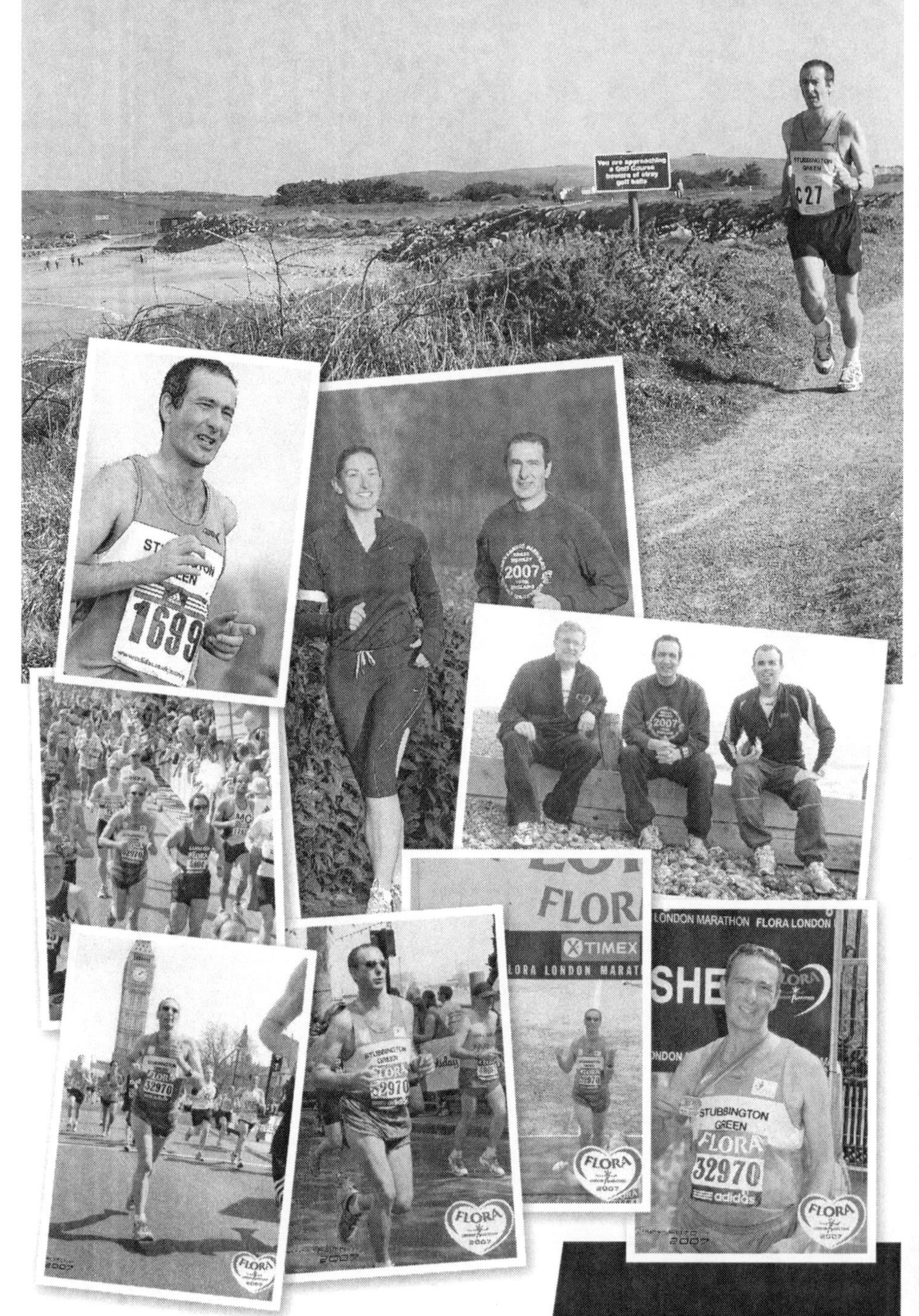
STUBBINGTON GREEN
C27
1699
2007
FLORA
TIMEX
LONDON MARATHON FLORA LONDON
STUBBINGTON GREEN
FLORA
32970
adidas

APRIL

17. Worthing 20 @ Worthing, West Sussex.

RUNNING the London Marathon is a bit like taking your car over 26 miles of speed bumps; you know the journey is going to be long and bloody uncomfortable, and though certain of reaching your destination, it's a lottery what will be hanging on at the end!

With two capital marathon capers under my belt in 2001 and 2004, I approached April with a huge amount of apprehension. Sunday, April 23rd and the Flora London Marathon hung over my head menacingly like a Damocles' Sword. Or put another way, I was now in the dentist's waiting room about to be summoned for root canal surgery after being told by a pretty receptionist that they've run out of anaesthetic.

In 2001, I got round the marathon course on a wing and a prayer with very little training, finishing in just over four hours. The biggest mistake I made then was to reach out and grab some sweets that were being handed out by kind folk as runners weaved their way around Canary Wharf, only to stuff a handful of vaseline into my mouth! No amount of water or trying to spit the stuff out would remove the bitter taste and texture.

Three years later, I had trained properly as the race became a ding-dong battle between myself and the model Nell McAndrew. She was accompanied by two barrel-chested minders. Everywhere we went a huge roar followed Nell sporting a tight-fitting outfit with barely any sweat dripping off that gorgeous figure. I looked like a poor man's Worzel Gummidge in a rain shower, and it was raining hard that Sunday morning in 2004.

We were going at a fair pace too at just over seven-and-a-half minute a mile pace, which was not hanging around. I had opened up a slight gap over Nell when, at 21 miles, my body hit the infamous wall. The wall is a fancy dan runner's term for what the men in white coats call glycogen depletion. Glycogen is your muscles' preferred fuel for aerobic exercise, so when runners "hit the wall" they have depleted their glycogen stores and have to rely increasingly on fat as a fuel source. When you have to burn more fat to keep going, you slow, and in some cases you stop. And even when you don't stop, you may run abnormally which can cause extra soreness in your muscles. Back in 2004, I was hallucinating.

As we headed through Wapping and past Tower Hill tube station I wanted someone to turn down the volume from the enthusiastic crowds who lined the route. This was a mini hell where I was being tormented by the demons of doubt imploring me to stop. My body had run out of fuel. I was cold, I was wet, I was hurting. All I could think was of Lance Armstrong, the seven-time Tour de France winner who had overcome cancer and stared death in the face to become one of the greatest cyclists of all time. His mantra is "pain is temporary, quitting is forever" which I kept reminding myself of; there was no way I was going to throw in the towel now. Amazingly, thanks to bloody mindedness plus stuffing down a combination of jelly babies and sports drinks, I beat the demons. Though my race pace slowed considerably I crossed the finish line in a respectable time of 3 hours and 19 minutes, just three minutes ahead of Nell and her muscular entourage.

I explain this as a backdrop to 2007. The expectation of the pain of the London Marathon had not diminished. As an occasional reminder I had kept some of the post-race marathon photographs from 2004 when I looked like the mime artist Marcel Marceau. My face was as white as a sheet and when I met my dad at the assembly point in Horse Guards Parade, I told him: "never again"!! Isn't that what Steve Redgrave once said after his fourth rowing gold medal?

So to revisit the marathon a further three years' later was sheer lunacy, especially with the very real possibility of picking up a long-term injury which could finish off the project. It would only take one nasty achilles or hamstring tear to kill off everything I had been working for. Yet running the London Marathon was a necessary part of the book. How could you write about running and racing around the British Isles without taking part in the most famous race of all? It would be like climbing the Three Peaks only to miss out on Snowdon or embarking on a culinary tour of Britain and ignoring McDonald's.

It was those haunting thoughts and painful memories of 2004 which had nagged in the back of my mind coming into April. This was my make or break month. I was also panicking slightly too.

Originally I had planned to head north on April Fool's Day to compete in the Baildon Boundary Half Marathon in Shipton. Organised by Baildon Runners in aid of a childhood cancer charity, Candlelighters, and Joel Harrison, a local boy who suffers from epilepsy and cerebral palsy, this is a very pretty run over the picturesque North Yorkshire countryside taking in woods, canal towpaths, and moors.

In fact the race route passes the original film site of Emmerdale's Woolpack pub, and heads through the Victorian village of Salts Mill on the edge of Saltaire which was designated a World Heritage site in December 2001. Later still, you run on the sandy gallops where Harvey Smith, the showjumper and racehorse trainer, exercises his horses, and within the first mile the course goes right past the entrance to the farmhouse belonging to Yorkshire and England cricketer, Matthew Hoggard! Truly a sightseers' paradise! But I still couldn't be persuaded to make the pilgrimage north because this was a half marathon and just 13 miles – ONLY 13 miles! I needed a 20-miler, vital miles in the bank and psychologically an important landmark to reach. After all, nail 20 miles three weeks before London, and it was only another six miles for the full marathon distance. So instead I joined Nick Kimber and Marcus Lee, two friends from Stubbington Green Runners, for the short drive along the coast to West Sussex for the Worthing 20.

The race was four very dull windswept laps on a course which looped along the shoreline looking out onto the English Channel and into the town of Goring. The beauty of the multi-lap course was that by the third lap I was overtaking the back markers and a succession of slower runners which eased the boredom factor. A time of 2 hours 33 minutes was a case of job done. The only side-effects were a minging headache and an embarrassing complaint of runner's nipple caused by my vest rubbing against my chest. Blood was smeared in two spots over the new and previously unwashed vest as if I'd been shot. The reason was that a few weeks earlier I'd had some white vests made especially for the challenge. This was one of the first outings for the garment which carried sponsors' logos plus branding on the back for the Hampshire Autistic Society.

If the project was about running alone it would be simple, but it was more than that. It was about raising both money and boosting the profile of autism, particularly the Hampshire Autistic Society. A weekly page in the Southern Daily Echo, plus a regular internet blog on the newspaper's website was generating good publicity for the cause. Thanks to sending off a string of e-mails to radio stations and newspapers around the UK, wherever I travelled I picked up some good media coverage.

The London Marathon, however, was a good hook for much of that publicity, and in the weeks leading up to April 23rd I was devoting a fair amount of time to interviews for newspapers, local radio, websites, and television. It was rewarding. Five minutes on BBC South Today, the regional evening TV programme for the south coast, provided vital airtime. The film clip, put together by a good journalism colleague of mine, Tony Husband, carried an interview plus images of myself, Ross and my eldest son Micah prancing on a trampoline in our back garden. It wasn't about massaging my huge ego, but providing vital platforms to talk about the year-long running adventure and about autism. It was getting the message through by beaming images of Ross into people's homes that this was the reality of autism – cruel, quiet, and complicated. Weeks and months later, it was amazing to discover the number of people who had seen that three minute film clip when the message about what I was doing and why had really hit home.

Also, by talking about the project it put the task into perspective. For the first time, the reality of what I was setting out to achieve, the size of the task and how momentous the outcome would be caught me like someone switching on a light in a darkened room. In interviews, inevitably once I had explained the running part of the challenge, conversation would turn to Ross and the problems he and others face with autism. "How did you feel the day you discovered your son had autism?" asked the BBC Radio Solent presenter, Jon Cuthill, when I appeared on his morning show. "It was devastating," I replied. "It changed our lives forever, but with every challenge there is an opportunity, and here was an opportunity to look after Ross, to confront autism head on and to build a better life for him." I added: "Think of the potential of an autistic child like a wine bottle with the cork pushed in tightly. All that potential is contained within the liquid in the bottle and the challenge is to slowly let the cork out. It's unlikely you will ever fully release the cork, but maybe, just maybe and with patience, you might allow some of the wine to seep out and see some of that potential realised."

As I was talking it dawned on me that possibly, for the first time in my life, I was doing something valuable. Not necessarily life changing, but something which might make a difference. It sounds pious and pompous to write about it now, but these interviews and the coverage I was generating provided an enormous catalyst to what I was doing. Here I was using my profile and persuasion in the media and whatever energy there was in my legs to make a difference for autism.

Jon then switched tacks to launch into the running theme of his popular radio show which was generating huge numbers of listeners' phone calls; people's house names. "So, Dave, have you ever had a house name?" asked Jon. "Well, my first home was a little semi-detached place in Norfolk, lovely garden in a beautiful village and we called the house Pimple…because we picked a nice spot for it!" Boom boom!

The media bandwagon in the weeks leading up to the London Marathon moved onto an early morning assignation with the celebrated round-the-world sailor Dee Caffari for a seven-mile run from her home just outside of Southampton to her company's offices near Fareham.

Dee was training towards the London Marathon to raise money for the charity Sail4Cancer, and for me to meet her was a big moment. A TV crew was there along with a photographer from the Daily Echo to capture the moment. I was in awe of Dee, an inspirational lady who, in May 2006, became the first woman to circumnavigate the globe the "wrong way" against the prevailing winds and currents, solo and non-stop. I could not imagine anything worse than hunkered down in the claustrophobic cabin of a yacht in the middle of a storm in the Southern Oceans; alone, exposed, and extremely vulnerable.

"Running, by far, is the furthest from my comfort zone that I have ever been," explained Dee. "It's like learning a new skill. For me, it is setting myself another challenge which I am taking step by step." As we passed the rush hour traffic we chatted of her previous life as a school teacher before she took a leap of faith to enter the world of sailing. She described what it was like to be alone on a yacht being battered by storms – "You just say to yourself this can't go on forever" adding that the key was having self-belief and an ability to face your fears. Dee's philosophy is: "We can do more than we think we can – we just have to dare to dream." Three weeks later, Dee completed the marathon in 7 hours and 20 minutes. It hurt, she was reduced at one stage to walking, but through dogged determination she fulfilled that dream.

18-21 Guernsey Easter Running Festival.

GUERNSEY was the next stop on the agenda. Two years earlier I had slagged off the Channel Island in a newspaper article. I had described Guernsey as boring and the locals dull and humourless after a dreary, watching paint dry Easter weekend in fogbound St Peter Port. The article had been picked up by the Guernsey Press prompting plenty of animated discussion.

I wondered whether this year I would be stopped at the airport's passport control with my dodgy Crimewatch photograph and the offending newspaper article pinned up in the officer's kiosk. Fortunately, a combination of unwashed hair, shabby clothing, Groucho Marx glasses and fake moustache, plus walking through customs glued to a copy of FHM did the trick since no-one raised an eyebrow. The short flight from Southampton to Guernsey wasn't without incident, though, because as the Flybe plane descended towards the runway, it had to pull out at the last minute because of another plane on the runway! Nice one!

This was another Easter weekend and a running festival organised by the island's athletics club made up of four races in four days. But this was not the Guernsey I had remembered. The weather was spectacular; bright sunshine and blue skies throughout the weekend. This was Guernsey, packed into 25 square miles, dressed in its finest garments, not in its ruffled bedclothes of a couple of years previously. The rocky coastline is dotted with the history of this fair isle; of the Napoloeonic whitewashed Martello Towers, and the

German gun emplacements, a reminder of the time more than 60 years ago when the Nazi jackboot landed on British soil. The pace of life is leisurely and so different to mainland Britain. In fact Guernsey is more akin to France just 60 miles distant, marked by the French place names, the 35mph speed limit and chequered yellow box junctions, the blue letter boxes and its own currency.

After each day's racing in the morning, Liz and I would head for a sun-kissed beach – there are more than two dozen in Guernsey - to relax in the afternoon and bronze our golden torsos – well, Liz did the bikini and sun lotion bit, I was left to wrestle with marking exam papers, testing journalists on the finer points of law and common sense, which was palpably lacking in quite a few of the offerings.

As for the running, it was as hot as the unseasonable Easter weather. Four races dotted about the island made up of the Heathspan 10km race on Good Friday from Rovers AC Football Club in Port Soif, the Keith Falla Memorial 4.75 mile cross country race at Les Amarreurs to the north of Guernsey on Saturday, and then back there on Easter Sunday for a 4x2 mile cross country relay.

The finale to the festival, which was in its 26th year, was the Heathspan Half Marathon starting in St Peter Port, heading along the coast road to the district of Vale and back to the capital. We had an exiled Zimbabwean, Williard Chinhanhu, now based in Poole, Dorset, who blasted away the opposition, a Kenyan, Guernsey's top middle distance runner, and among the women one youngster from the Aldershot, Farnham & District Club who is sure to be a star of tomorrow. Remember the name Steph Twell, then just 17, and already a European Junior Cross Country Champion.

Here's a stark contrast. Steph and UK Athletics performance coach, Mick Woods, were leaning against a car parked next to mine in the Albert Pier Car Park in St Peter Port on the final day of competition. The half marathon was half an hour away. I was going through my amateur routine of a pre-race chocolate bar, sports drink, checking the weekend's football results in the paper, singing along to some cheesy 80s hits on the Ipod and going through the motions of a couple of flimsy stretching exercises. Steph, meanwhile, was getting a full low down from Mick; stretches, race tactics, race mindset, as she downed a sports drink while listening intently. She had the body of a gazelle, the stamina of an ox, and a youthfulness to envy. A couple of hours later, Steph smashed a 25-year record by breaking the UK junior half marathon record in 1 hour 17 minutes 27 seconds in her first outing at that distance and in pretty sticky temperatures. Just incredible! I was more than 20 minutes or more than two-and-a-half miles behind Steph finishing in 1:38.27.

For the record, while Steph was tearing up the Guernsey countryside, I was meandering my way through a 10km in 44 minutes 9 seconds, the cross country in 34 minutes 48 seconds and ran the third leg of the cross country in 13 minutes 45 seconds. All in all 26 miles of running, marathon distance, another step towards London, and 21 races down in the 80 race challenge.

22. Flitwick 10k @ Flitwick, Bedfordshire.

CONVENTIONAL wisdom is that at least two weeks before the marathon you should allow the body to rest – or taper, which is the buzz word. I first came across the word taper when I was writing about swimming for a newspaper in Portsmouth.

The Olympic silver medallist, Sharron Davies, was on the Portsmouth swim team at the time and she first told me about this tapering malarkey. How swimmers would prepare for competition by reining back on their early morning training which ordinarily consisted of swimming a masochistic 70km a week at 5.30am and again at teatime. And then we talked shaving! "It cuts down resistance in the water. When you're swimming in championships, tenths of a second count," Sharron once told me. I had a saucy follow-up question about shaving which only a bloke would ask and which I was dying to answer Sharron, but I didn't have the bottle. She was taller than me!

So with that in mind I came up with the idea of a pre-London Marathon Wax & Go. I decided to get my legs waxed on the Monday before the big day; good publicity and a great vehicle for raising some valuable sponsorship from friends, family and workmates.

The girls at the Hampshire Autistic Society managed to find a salon willing to perform the dirty deed. Back in February I had popped down to Elysium Health & Beauty in Whiteley near Fareham for a test waxing to check my pain tolerance as well as to see if there was any nasty after effects. There weren't! So come the big day, I turned up bright and early to meet the salon's owner, Angela Anderson, ready and willing for my legs to face her waxing strips. Friends had suggested waxing other regions of my body, including the infamous back, crack and sack, but Angela was unwilling to delve into parts other women cannot reach and, out of good taste, she declined the opportunity!

I was sat on a couch in the shop window with Angela waxing lyrical and a photographer getting me to pose for pictures in various states of agony. I had carried one sick thought of keeping the hairs, sticking them in a jam jar and auctioning them on eBay. After all, if people were prepared to part with good money for a Tesco shopping bag, why not a jam jar of someone's leg hair?! Commonsense prevailed, and that madcap publicity stunt was ditched in the salon bin.

The waxing itself passed off well. It wasn't too painful, except for some delicate areas around the bikini wax line – not that I wear a bikini or am prepared to admit the fact – and also around the hamstrings. By the end of the session I looked like a plucked chicken, and once I had swapped the shorts for a pair of trousers, the sensation was very unusual. For the next few days, my legs felt wet as they brushed against my trousers. Requests to show and tell proved popular as over the next few weeks sponsors demanded proof that the deed had indeed been done and more than £2,000 was raised for the Hampshire Autistic Society.

In common with the tapering theme, the final race before the marathon was a gentle 10km run in Flitwick, Bedfordshire. There I caught up with my oldest school friend, Kevin Holley. We'd grown up in the west London town of Ruislip, best known for a spy scandal in the 1960s, Leslie Thomas's "Tropic of Ruislip" – and wife swapping, apparently, but little else. It was typical middle class London suburbia. We went to primary school together, passed the 11 plus together, endured the trials, tribulations and tears of various pathetic attempts at teenage romances with a string of contenders, gone through O levels and A levels at the local Grammar School, and been best man at each others weddings.

Now aged 44, we were both separated from our wives, both losing our hair and putting on a fair bit of weight around the middle. Kevin was a classic sports skiver at school. He would conjure up any excuse to avoid PE. Those were the days when Wednesday afternoons were a choice of rugby or cross country, and on really bad weather days, British Bulldog in the gym! The only sport Kevin did enjoy was sailing when I was occasionally press-ganged into crewing the Mirror dinghy he kept at the Ruislip Lido. He always chose god-forsaken cold days for me to sit at the front of the boat, pulling the ropes – or sheets to use the technical term - while making sure the Spinnaker had the right shape. Boy was it boring and my bottom ached after two hours sitting on the lake with barely a breath of wind blowing!

Now in middle age, Kevin had found golf and, in recent years, running. Running and Kevin seemed the most unlikeliest of bedfellows, but the man had completed a marathon, he'd even finished a triathlon and here was his way of stepping off the hamster wheel of life by doing something completely different. April was enjoying something of a sunfest, and this was another beautiful day for a run over a fast and undulating course in the heart of the Bedfordshire countryside.

The Flitwick 10k formed part of the Bedfordshire 10km Championships, a well run and organised event staged by the Ampthill & Flitwick Flyers, whose race director, Keith Morgan, kindly gave me a free entry to the run. I knew Kevin wouldn't be fast, and that was perfect. We jogged at the sort of pace where conversation comes easily, catching up on the latest news and gossip. It was a very pleasant run out of Flitwick, through the village of Steppingley, skirting the M1 at half way, and then easing back into the village in a leisurely time of 51 minutes 57 seconds.

23 Flora London Marathon.

AND so the week of the marathon beckoned. Waxing on the Monday, and then work formed the sideshow to the build-up. Concentrating on anything but the race was difficult. After Flitwick I had decided not to run again before the marathon to completely rest.

Throughout the year I had been working closely with a dietician based at Southampton General Hospital, Jenny Davies, who had outlined a programme of eating and drinking for all my races. She wanted me to cut out the fats, snack more efficiently, and drink more liquid. When Jenny suggested in her lilting Welsh tones that I should be drinking up to five litres of liquid a day, I almost fell of my chair. "I'll need to start wearing nappies or have a catheter fitted," I pleaded. "You just need to get used to it," replied Jenny. So for the past month I had been on this new regime. Not quite five litres a day, but close to three litres, and I was peeing for Britain! If peeing was an Olympic sport based on volume, shortlist me as a contender for London in 2012!

"Look at the colour of your urine," Jenny once told me. "You are aiming for it to be straw-like in colour - the lighter the better. Tea is not an ideal re-hydration fluid. Better ones would be water, diluted squash, diluted fruit juice, sports drinks (hypotonic or isotonic). Try and avoid fizzy drinks like coca-cola and lemonade.

"The other thing you need to increase in your diet is the amount of carbohydrate. However, don't skimp on your bread, potatoes, rice, pasta, crackers etc. and also take on board sugary, but low fat carbohydrates like jelly babies, fruit pastilles, boiled sweets, fruit - including dried fruit." It was a lot to take in as Jenny gave me a comprehensive list of snacks which I could and could not eat.

However come the week of the marathon I felt unwell. My stomach was sore and ached. I feared that I might have picked up a urinary infection. Tests with the doctors looked for an infection, even a grumbling appendix, but found none. The doctor wondered if it was simply a case of nerves – it probably was. To use a modern colloquial term, I was bricking it big time.

Come Saturday, the day before the race, the top athletes would have been holed up at their luxurious five-star London hotel, treated to massages, eaten specially chosen foods and enjoyed the pampering of a Hollywood star. Me? No way! I was holed up in court room number 4 at Portsmouth Magistrates' Court on Saturday morning, a bottle of water secretly tucked beside my leg, and a bag of jelly babies sat in my suit pocket.

Besides working as a journalist, my other job is as a Justice of the Peace serving the South-East Hampshire bench in Portsmouth. The criminal justice system fascinates me. Bizarre, I know, but I wanted to learn more about crime – not to participate in it, but to find out what prompts those to offend, if it is possible to turn someone from a pattern of crime, and what was being done to those who are convicted – rehabilitation, punishment, reparation? Now in my third year as a magistrate, I was sitting as part of a bench of three twice a month. It's unpaid, it's unglamorous, but it is worthwhile.

Ever so often, we are occasionally called upon to sit on a Saturday court, and it was my turn. On the eve of the London Marathon we had five cases, all prisoners who had been remanded in prison on various charges of assault, theft and one of cultivating cannabis plants. None of the cases could be heard in full, the question for myself and two other colleagues was whether, having already spent at least a night in a prison cell, these men should be given their freedom and released on bail before their cases would finally be heard in court. To be honest, despite the submissions of their solicitors, the decisions weren't difficult. For reasons such as a risk of reoffending, threatening witnesses and even the possibility of fleeing the country, one by one bail was refused, and from the dock 30 foot away, they were handcuffed by the warders, led away down the steps to the cells below and in the van back to Winchester Prison.

One close cropped, scowling defendant gestured with his cupped hands something about an anchor as the chairman read out the pronouncement that bail had been refused. I looked at a print out of his previous convictions. This man was just a month older than me, he had been in trouble with the police since the age of 13 and had spent almost 15 years behind bars in that time. He was 44, but his gaunt face, deep haunting eyes, and sallow complexion, added at least 10 years onto that age. What a waste of a life.

For the final part of the morning, I was ushered off to a side room on my own where I was confronted with a court clerk and a social worker. The issue at hand was to decide whether to section under the Mental Health Act a person who was proving a danger to himself and the public. This was playing God time, with one swift signature having the ability to take away someone's liberty. It is a responsibility you don't treat lightly. The evidence was compelling, the answers to my questions honest and to the point. I signed the paper, walked out of the room, knowing that later that afternoon police would pick up this man and escort him from his home to a secure mental hospital.

From the magistrates' court it was straight on a train from Southampton to London with Liz and an overnight stay at the Novotel near Lambeth Palace. We'd hitched up with one of the marathon tour companies who lay on food in the evening, accommodation, a 6am pre-race breakfast and then a coach to take you to the start at Blackheath.

Friends were catching a 5am coach from the south coast to get to the south-east London, but I did not want to be sat on a bus for a long time hurtling to the toilet every five minutes. The pre-night stay, though not cheap, had worked well in the past. Well, except for the time three years ago when I stayed at an hotel on the Strand sharing a room with a runner who was prancing around practising wearing a four-foot tall plywood banner advertising the name of his company from Bolton – and asking whether I thought it was over the top?!! Then in 2001, I stayed in another hotel the night before the London Marathon hoping for a good night's sleep only to be woken by the joyful sounds of a passionate couple engaged in several rounds of horizontal dancing on a creaky bed. Jesus was the name of the bloke, or that was what the woman was screaming at the top of her voice.

Preparation was everything – running was the easy part!

I slept well. Any thoughts of Liz and I dancing the night Fandango were swiftly cast to one side. There are several schools of thought about pre-race nookie and running - a necessary release of pent up energy and frustration and a perfect way to relax before the big event – or an unnecessary draining of energy at a time when you needed to save all the calories. Maybe I should have asked Sharron Davies the question when we were talking about shaving and tapering!

Come the morning itself, the weather was bright and sunny. Two coaches lined up outside the hotel at 7am after we had breakfasted – porridge, banana and a glass of orange juice. I was as nervous as a kitten sat on the coach listening to my iPod as we set off to Blackheath, working through a race plan in my head. Twenty minutes into the ride and I was busting for the toilet and we had only just reached Streatham. Another runner had tried the on-coach loo, but it wasn't working. The journey across London seemed to take an age and progressively my bladder was bursting. I was panicking trying all sorts of distraction therapies to take my mind off the dilemma. I wanted desperately to get off the bus. I had a half empty bottle of water in my rucksack and thoughts turned to relieving myself in the bottle! The journey took well over an hour as traffic crawled round Greenwich and to our destination. I shot off the bus, crouched behind some parked cars and the relief was overwhelming. In life there are several events which can be classed as supreme moments of relief – a desperately-needed constitutional is one, a comfy bed and a soft pillow is another, a cold fizzy drink on a boiling hot day or a piece of chocolate to settle an empty stomach are others which have that "argh, boy did I need that" moment.

It was hot, very hot and it was only 8.45am. I was also very late. I had hoped to be at the Blackheath by 8am, a good hour and three quarters from the start to prepare properly. Now, at the green start, the smallest of the three London Marathon starts, which hosts the celebrities, media runners and those with "good for age" times, I felt rushed. I plonked myself on the grass next to an old fella who was smearing vaseline on his eyebrows. "What are you doing that for?" I asked. "It stops the sweat getting in your eyes," he replied. "It's a useful trick and works every time." I decided to do the same as we chatted. The guy was a veteran of 26 London Marathons. He kept coming back every year as a pilgrimage. His whole year was built around this one day in April. "It's going to be hot today," he warned. "You be careful out there and make sure you drink properly. I think there could be some problems for quite a few runners."

I stuffed down another banana and a sports drink, swallowed a couple of Immodium tablets to avoid any calls of nature on route, took a Voltarol pain relieving tablet and shoved another in my pocket. Once changed, I handed my bag to one of the volunteers standing by a fleet of lorries which would take the tens of thousands of white London Marathon bags to the finish in The Mall.

The butterflies were really working overtime as we lined up in our starting pens; the key was to get the butterflies flying in formation. I found a friend, Mary Picksley, who I had run with two months earlier in Stamford and who had agreed to run with me today. Mary was in her late 50s, from Sheffield, and who had once finished third in her class at the London Marathon. When we had talked shortly before the marathon, Mary had hinted about the possibility of tackling an age group record of 3 hours 8 minutes for the marathon. But looking up at the cloudless blue sky, and feeling the heat of the burning sun on our faces, we knew that this was a non-starter. Even without the knotted handkerchief, I looked like a tourist on Blackpool beach, coated in suntan lotion and sporting dark glasses. No records, instead, we agreed would pace each other and use our experience to work our way through the crowds.

The start was congested. The slower celebrities always get to the front as I side-stepped my way first past Floella Benjamin and then Gordon Ramsey. You could barely run, you were trotting shoulder to shoulder with other runners. One unfortunate soul missed a traffic island – heaven knows how – and was sent spinning to the floor, another tripped over a speed bump and was saved from falling flat on his face by a runner with an outstretched arm.

The first mile Mary and I ran through in 7 minutes 47 seconds – we were looking at 7 minutes 30 seconds a mile pacing – but very soon we settled into a comfortable rhythm picking our way through the field as the green start merged with runners from the blue start on Shooter's Hill Road and then with the red start three miles into the race by Woolwich Dockyard. The noise was incredible; a non-stop din of cheering crowds, live bands playing by the side of the road, music pumping out of speakers and DJs screaming choruses of encouragement. The feeling of well-bring is immense. Running is music to the soul and in a world of greed and frequent selfishness, the London Marathon restores your faith in human nature. Never mind the millions of pounds which were being raised for charity, it is man's support for fellow man in adverse conditions which brings raw emotions to the surface. It is why the London Marathon is so special and where, when your muscles are hurting and your brain is screaming for you to slow down or stop, the atmosphere carries you on a wave of non-stop emotion.

From two miles on there were water stations at every mile with sports drinks available at every five. Learning from the mistakes of three years earlier, I knew that I had to stick to the plan of taking water at every other mile, and then listening to the words of Jenny Davies, the dietician, by taking as much of the Lucozade sports drink as I could. The orange flavoured Isotonic drinks are good for replacing fluids and providing carbohydrate to fuel the muscles. The small 330ml packs being handed out at the marathon also contained some salt which, according to Jenny, would enhance the absorption and retention of fluid in your body. "If you want to avoid hitting the wall again then make sure you drink to replace the sweat you will lose and using the carbohydrate to replace energy stores," said Jenny. It was the best piece of advice she could give and ultimately saved me on the day. I slowed at the water stations and jogged to take on the fluid. Never mind I was being passed by other runners, some carrying camel sacks on their backs with water tubes leading to their mouths, others carrying belts around their waists replete with liquid carriers and a ribbon of high-energy gels. Bizarrely, some of them were so packaged to the gunnels they looked like suicide bombers! What I knew is that with my careful drinks strategy, I would catch them.

Mary was surprisingly struggling. Later I was to learn that she had bought a new pair of socks and was wearing them for the first time in the race. As a result she was slowing with an achilles problem. I held back trying to encourage her, although the temptation was to push on. Landmarks came and went; the Cutty Sark at Greenwich, and then we swept under Tower Bridge with huge crowds gathered on both sides. The noise reverberated around the metal structure of this historic bridge, the hairs stood on the back of your neck. We were 13 miles in and half way, and Mary was hurting. We had agreed we would pace each other, but if one was feeling stronger then they should not feel guilty and go at their own pace. Just as I could see the leading men pass on the opposite side of the Highway, eight miles ahead, I went for it and pushed on. Seeing the top Kenyans was dumbfounding. Their feet floated on the tarmac, breezing past on the opposite side of the road with an economy of effort as if going for a Sunday stroll. Facing them on the other side of the carriageway was a tide of weary runners casting envious looks at those born with an amazing god-given talent.

Feeling a little heavy legged, I surprised myself by picking up the pace to pass runners regularly. Liz should have been stood somewhere around the 14-mile mark with a bag of goodies, but was lost in the huge crowds. At 15 miles, the race moved into the Isle of Dogs which gets quite claustrophobic at times. It was then that the heavy aching legs became painful. I had 11 miles to go, and though the top half of my body was fine and fit, the bottom half was hurting. I took another painkiller as I could feel the pace slowing, but resolutely I stuck to the drinks strategy. Every mile passed became another victory. I spotted my dad on Poplar High Street at mile 20 with a plastic bag containing jelly babies and Kendal Mint Cake – wonderful! That was my treat for every mile passed.

Runners were falling by the wayside, many walking in the middle of the road, some bent over crash barriers exhausted. One man collapsed in front of me, his knees buckling before falling to the ground. Several members of the crowd rushed out to help him. The heat was unrelenting. It was humid and sticky. There was no breeze and everyone was burning up. Another white-faced victim sat by the side of the road spewing her guts out, a third was being tended by St John Ambulance on a stretcher with an oxygen mask over his mouth and his body wrapped in an aluminium sheet. It was distressing to witness these casualties of a race. It was like a war zone.

I later heard that a Stubbington team-mate of mine, who I had seen tearing past me at the five-mile mark, had collapsed exhausted just a few hundred yards from the finish. Graham Bell, who was raising money for the Parkinson's Disease Society, was pulled out of the race within 500 yards of the finish. After three attempts by St John's Ambulance to get Graham on his feet, he was counted out on the fourth collapse. "I got to 20 miles bang on seven minute miling," said Graham later. "Then it went all to pot. I struggled through mile by mile until mile 25, and then it went wrong big time. I spent two hours in recovery at the St John's base outside Buckingham Palace, and two hours at University College Hospital. I was feeling a bit sore and a bit of a prat."

Meanwhile for me, the demons of doubt lingered in the background, but having conquered them once three years ago, they weren't even in the race this time. This was a race of attrition, a battle where there was only going to be one winner. I was counting to myself, singing tunes in my head, trying to switch off from the occasion by allowing it to wash over me. Past Tower Hill, sweeping by London Bridge and Blackfriars, through Charing Cross at 25 miles and along the Embankment.

Just before we turned at the Palace of Westminster into Birdcage Walk I spotted a friend of mine Tex Dallas. It was amazing that I was able to pick him out from the throng. Tex had been a great source of inspiration for my previous two marathons, and for the first one in 2001 we had trained together. Tex spotted me and shouted "Go on Davy boy, you can do this." We high-fived, and that was the spur I needed. Sod the pain, sod the whinging, get on and finish the bloody job. I gritted my teeth and pushed on for that final mile.

The crowds were now larger and louder than ever. Buckingham Palace soared into view at mile 26, a swift right turn and into the Mall where the finishing line loomed ahead. Thank god I was wearing sunglasses because I was bawling my eyes out for those final couple of hundred yards. That was my emotional relief, the end of this particular journey which I had survived. I punched the air with absolute pleasure when I crossed the finishing line – 3 hours 29 minutes and 24 seconds. Perfect!

That was hard. The World Cup rugby star, Matt Dawson who took part was later to describe conditions as "brutal" on a day when temperatures reached 21c. Gordon Ramsey said: "It was like running in a desert today. They were dropping like flies." St John Ambulance treated 5,032 people and of those 73 were sent to hospital for further treatment.

Sadly 22-year-old fitness instructor David Rogers from Milton Keynes collapsed during the race and later died due to hyponatraemia. The condition, a lack of sodium in his body, can be caused by drinking too much water. It was a jarring thought because here was a young man who had shared the same epic and long journey as myself and the other 35,000 souls who lined up at Blackheath on April 23rd, who battled through the most extreme conditions for marathon running, who courageously finished, but who was unable to savour the magnificent achievement. I grabbed hold of the chunky medal with its green, red, blue and yellow ribbon and wore it with pride all the way home.

24. Horton Bull Run @ Chipping Sodbury, Bristol.

THANKFULLY, the marathon had left very little damage. I was sore and both my hamstrings and quadriceps ached, but there were no major muscular issues. Twenty four hours after the race I had an hour-long massage from physiotherapist Mark Diment when he professed there was nothing to worry about. "You're in bloody good shape for a man who's just run 26 miles," was his verdict. For the next couple of days walking down stairs was a bit of an issue, but by the Thursday my body was feeling good, and for anyone who wanted to see, both the medal and shaven legs were on parade in the office – in return for suitable sponsorship.

I wanted to wind down the month with a quiet race, nothing too hard or serious, and so a trip to the Cotswolds the weekend after the London Marathon provided the perfect antidote.

The Bull Run 4 takes place in the small village of Horton in Gloucestershire. Bob Bell, the club chairman with the delightfully named Hogweed Trotters, who organise the race, joked: "We don't get much happening round these parts. In fact besides the race, the next most exciting event is the annual dry stone wall building competition. Oh, and we had a pretty juicy murder here back in the 1990s."

The Horton Bull Run was originally a six-mile race and was first staged 23 years ago. Then the start was led off by the Green Goddess, Diana Moran. Since then, the Hogweed Trotters have reduced the distance to make it an easy introduction to running for many people.

The race was a four-mile run besides the Cotswold Escarpment along tiny country lanes. I was surprised by how many young children were taking part. But this was a fantastic day out in some beautiful countryside, with bacon butties and steaming cups of tea being served from the village hall kitchen besides posters advertising auditions for this year's village panto, Cinderella. Everyone was so friendly, it was such a small and intimate race and such a contrast from a week earlier.

It was a measure of the standard of entry for the race that from an entry of 200 I finished a nose-bleeding high 27th and fourth in my age group. This was a lovely gentle run with a couple of testing hills thrown in.

At one stage I was passed by a 15-year-old wearing an England football shirt with the words Michael Owen on the back. The humiliation of it! I was a London Marathon runner, a supreme athlete, being made mince-meat of by someone almost three times younger than me. So I eased up alongside him and said: "You okay? You do know it's two laps, don't you?!!" The kid look bemused and I seized on that moment's hesitation to forge ahead and leave the youngster trailing in my wake. Eat dust you whippersnapper! I wasn't proud of that cruel bit of gamesmanship, but I'll be darned if I was allowing a 15-year-old boy to beat me in a sprint finish!

The main point for me was that I had survived April, and got through the tricky test of the London Marathon. Four months down, 24 races completed, hey, the only way is up!

"Running is like mouthwash; if you can feel the burn, it's working."

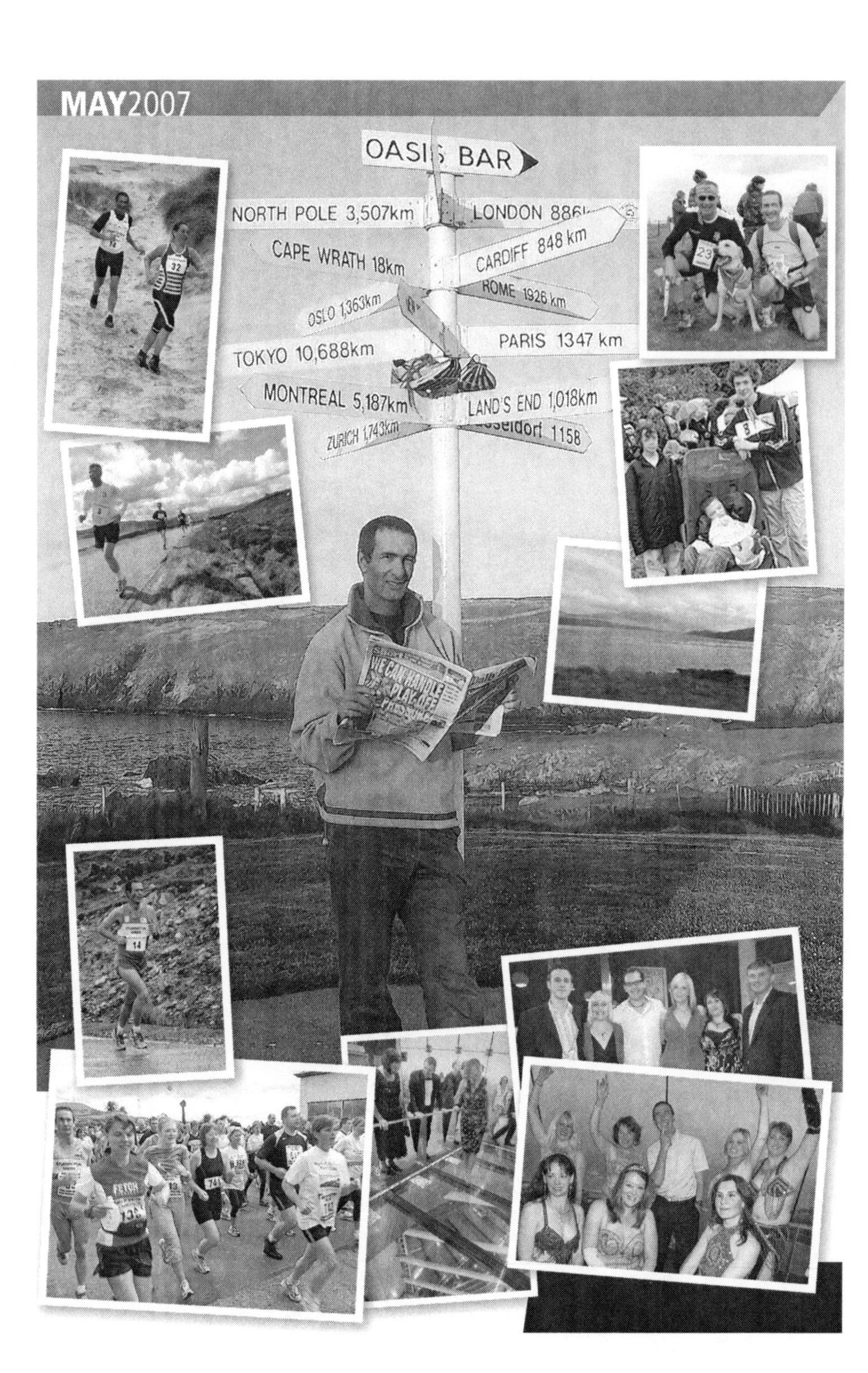
MAY2007
OASIS BAR
NORTH POLE 3,507km
LONDON 886
CAPE WRATH 18km
CARDIFF 848 km
OSLO 1,363km
ROME 1926 km
TOKYO 10,688km
PARIS 1347 km
MONTREAL 5,187km
LAND'S END 1,018km
ZURICH 1,743km
1158

MAY

25. Dudley Kingswinford 10k @ Dudley, West Midlands.

NEIL FEREDAY and the Dudley Kingswinford 10k have a special bond stretching back more than 20 years. The 53-year-old lorry driver from Tipton in the West Midlands hasn't missed a single DK10k – widely regarded as the London Marathon of 10km evening races. "I just love this race. It's my club race and every year I make a point of taking part," explained Neil, who had run all the previous 21 10ks with a best time of 34 minutes 32 seconds at the very first race.

The West Midlands town lies in the heart of the Black Country able to trace its history back to Roman times. And the DK10k is regarded as one of the premier running events in the region, the largest midweek evening race in the midlands having been first staged in 1986 and cancelled just once, in 2001, because of the foot and mouth outbreak. There were more than 1,000 runners at the Dudley Kingswinford Running Club for the 22nd running of the race served up on a beautiful sun-kissed early summer's evening.

We met on a warm Wednesday evening at Dudley Kingswinford Rugby Club half an hour before race start. Neil wasn't a happy bunny. "I'm not feeling great," he confessed. "I've got a bit of a niggle with my hamstring which I picked up in training last week and if this wasn't the club 10km then I definitely wouldn't run. I'm not going to miss this one, no way. I've not even thought about sitting this one out." True to form, the muscular runner was there on the start line wearing the light and dark blue hooped running vest of Dudley Kingswinford Running Club, together with a natty pair of blue shorts to match, determined not to allow this amazing running streak to be broken.

"There is something very special about this club," explained Neil. "The race was begun by a guy called Dr Dick Blackburn, who is dead now, but who was one of the founders of the Dudley Kingswinford Running Club. Dick was an ex-rugby player and when he stopped playing he started a keep-fit class at a time when the marathon boom was taking hold. There were so many people interested in running that the club was started.

"The race has just grown in popularity over the years. I think it is so popular because this is one of the first 10k's of the season and we get runners from all the clubs in the area such as Tipton Harriers, Wolverhampton & Bilston taking part."

I don't know what it is about the brain and the body working in opposition, but they seem to have separate identities. I wanted a nice steady run in Dudley, but instead I blasted out of the blocks crashing through the first kilometre in just under four minutes, and by half way I was running 20 minutes for 5km. I was telling myself to slow down. I was barely a quarter of the way through the running challenge, I had a shed load of races lined up when my finishing time was irrelevant. But the body just kept pushing on the shoulders of other runners and then forging ahead along the quiet lanes around Kingswinford.

It was Neil, however, who put the brakes on. I spotted him just after the 5km mark and drew up alongside. He was struggling, his hamstring was hurting bad and I could tell by the look on his face that he was not wimping out. I decided to slow down and stick with Neil to get him to the finish. This was a wise move. We chatted for the second half of the race which seemed to flash by in a hurry as we ran to the finish together. "Running is a way of life for me," said Neil. "I'm stuck in traffic jams in my lorry during the day getting frustrated, in the evening I want to get out and run. It is a release."

Everyone seemed to know Neil as we picked our way up Little Check Hill. Friends were shouting encouragement, we ran past a throng of cheering people outside the Navigation Pub a mile from the finish which was bursting at the seams. Neil faced the prospect of a drive to Nottingham the following day when he knew his body was going to hurt after this run. The course was undulating with a couple of stiff climbs. At one of these, Neil explained that this was the route of their Boxing Day run, and at the top of the hill he pointed to the spot where he was always sick – usually through too much festive excess!

We had a pedal cycle escort towards the end of the race from one of Neil's mates as we strode out to the finish at the rugby club. We both clocked 45 minutes and one second for 10km to receive a lovely glass goblet at the end. For Neil, he said that running was about getting rid of the frustrations of lorry driving. He loves his sport, and I knew that the following day sat in his cab, he would be hurting! "Thanks mate," said Neil. "Thanks for pulling me through. How long will I continue running this race? I have no idea. It is becoming a bit of a personal quest."

For me, I was back in the office the following morning after driving back from Birmingham where a Post-It had been left on my desk asking me to call a Lloyd Scott. The name rang a bell, and then it tumbled. Lloyd is the lad who has made a habit of dressing up at the London Marathon. He's walked the course dressed in a 59kg deep sea diving suit, in a suit of armour, and this year I was standing next to him at the green start where he was dressed up as Indiana Jones, pulling behind this huge boulder. It took Lloyd the best part of 23 hours to complete the race raising money for the Unicorn Children's Theatre and First Step.

Throughout 2007 I had been writing a regular blog on the newspaper's website and a weekly column in the Southern Daily Echo about the challenge. In one of the articles I wrote after the London Marathon, I took a pop at Lloyd and some of the other cartoon caper characters who now took part in the race who, in my humble opinion, devalue the whole event. This year, for example, we had one guy running in slow motion, travelling three miles every 10 hours taking eight days to finish. Another walked backwards to set a world record. At times this showpiece in the running calendar has become nothing more than a glorified sponsored walk. For the tens of thousands of runners who complete the London Marathon it is the end of a six-month journey, of hard training runs on cold, dark nights or on windy wintry Sunday mornings, pounding the streets and the footpaths with the aim of running the magical distance of 26.2 miles. In my newspaper column, I wrote how I did not believe Lloyd's stunt to recreate the opening scene from the film Raiders Of The Lost Ark was in the spirit of what the London Marathon was all about.

Lo and behold, Lloyd, who lives in Rainham, Essex, saw the article after it was shown to him by a friend who'd been to a football match in Southampton. Lloyd was on the phone to complain about the piece. To be fair, what started as a heated exchange, ended on very friendly terms with Lloyd offering any help he could give to boost my fund-raising efforts. "I train just as hard for the marathon as any other runner," explained Lloyd, who pointed out how he too had to focus on diet and hydration. However he explained that his progress at the London Marathon had been hampered by health and safety regulations. He finished his race at 8am on the Monday morning, having taken an overnight rest on the Sunday and then recommenced at 2am so as to beat the rush hour traffic. I have the utmost respect for Lloyd, the former fireman who was once diagnosed with chronic myeloid leukaemia and survived thanks to a bone marrow transplant. He has raised £5 million for cancer charities and was awarded an MBE in 2005. It was with a touch of irony that for the 2008 London Marathon, Lloyd completed the race dressed as a nine-foot high iron giant to raise money for an autism charity.

26 Round The Tree 3 @ Torrington, Devon.

THERE I was sat high on this hill looking down at the River Torridge snaking its way through the valley below, a sweeping vista across the Devon countryside bathed in warm Spring sunshine. This was the life, I thought, as I tucked into a steak and kidney pie and chips while nursing a cold can of full fat coca-cola just an hour before the race. Not your classic pre-race training diet, but good enough!

I was in Torrington in mid-Devon on a Friday evening for a race called Round The Tree 3. Great Torrington is situated high on the hill, and the race forms part of a weekend of May Day activities which also includes a carnival and maypole dancing.

The village had turned out in force for the race, which started and finished in the tiny market square. Drinkers from the Black Horse pub were watching with amusement at runners, some serious, and some in fancy dress, limbered up for the start of their races.

There were three races - one for boys, one for both girls and ladies, and then the men. I was feeling pretty tired come race time, not because of racing in Birmingham 48 hours earlier, but the previous evening I had hosted a fund-raising reception at the Spinnaker Tower in Portsmouth, which was sponsored by Haywood Office Services.

Sadly, the day of the event coincided with the funeral at Winchester Cathedral of the England footballer, Alan Ball, who had suddenly died of a heart attack a few weeks earlier aged 61. A neighbour of mine in the Hampshire village of Hook, I had known Alan for many years through work. He was a keen supporter of the Hampshire Autistic Society, and had agreed to help me that evening by attending the reception, where he had put up an auction prize. Despite Alan's death we still went ahead with the auction of a signed 1966 England World Cup framed photograph which raised a princely sum as the evening fetched a very handy £2,000 for the society. In fact, the reception went down really well, especially the scantily-clad belly dancers called Mystical Fusion who performed in a glass room, some 300 feet up with a spectacular view across the Solent, along with a magician and a fantastic singer called Amy Fern.

At the end of the evening I was asked to give a short speech about the challenge when I recalled a conversation I'd shared with the great adventurer, Sir Chay Blyth, a few years back. Life is about living on the edge, Sir Chay told me in the interview. My challenge happens to be running, his happened to be ocean sailing. This is a man who rowed across the Atlantic in a 20 foot Open Dory in 1966 with Captain John Ridgeway, and who in 1971 became the first person to sail non-stop westwards around the world against the prevailing winds and currents. A feat no one had ever previously attempted.

At the time of the interview a few years ago, Sir Chay was heading a business which, for the princely sum of £28,000, was offering people from all walks of life the opportunity to take a year out of the rat race to sail round the world the wrong way, as he did 30 years earlier. The opportunity came with a team of a 10 other sailors and a skipper aboard a 72-foot boat. Personally, I wouldn't choose to be thrown about the Southern Ocean cramped inside a steel-hulled yacht in growling, icy seas, just as others would baulk at the sadistic notion of running 26 miles and 385 yards. For me running is a release, a motivator, free-thinking time and an eternal challenge. It is a discipline, it is also obsessive. My bible is a running log book which records my daily mileage. It also acts as a confessional, plus a sobering reminder when that discipline slips and I fail to go for a run.

So I asked Sir Chay what made someone remortgage their home, leave their friends and family for 12 months and change their whole lifestyle for the sake of sailing round the world? He replied that life was about living on the edge. It was about pushing yourself to your limits both mentally and physically, so that come the time you get to meet your maker and look down at your crinkly toes, you can say you lived your life without regrets and you gave your best. I guess that's what I've been trying to do with this running challenge and this was the tale I told to the gathering at the Spinnaker Tower.

We didn't get clear of Portsmouth until gone midnight, I lost my ticket in the car park, and then I was back at work in the Southern Daily Echo building less than four hours later to oversee coverage of the local council elections. With just a few hours' sleep, and a slow four-hour drive on crowded single carriageway roads to Devon choking with May Bank Holiday traffic, I was wilting by the time I got to Great Torrington - hence the reason for the full fat coca-cola!

The Round The Tree race is believed to have started as early as the 1920s when it was always held on a Thursday evening. The original course went straight over the top of the common and through the River Torridge at Lady Island, over Mucksly Lane into the next field, around a tree and back along the same route to the finish. Runners would complete the race bruised, scratched and bleeding since there was no path to the common and so runners would take the shortest route. The prize for winning the race was the princely sum of 10 shillings.

For some reason, the race was stopped in the 1960s, though it is unclear precisely why. However the Round The Three 3 was reinstated 20 years later when a new course was set up, along with a tree following a course which continues to this day. When the tree died, runners ran around various objects on the course in place of a tree, but then two years ago a new tree was planted.

The race, organised by Torrington Athletic Club, was the wake-up call I needed. The men's field wasn't that big - maybe 70 or so, as we hurtled off down the hill, snaking around the village and towards the river. The descent was long and fast, yet any enjoyment was countered with the awful knowledge that we'd have a hard climb to the finish.

I paced the race quite comfortably, and soon began pulling back on some of the runners. The path uphill to Great Torrington was a gruelling climb. Half way up, a marshal shouted that the worst was over. She was wrong! We turned a corner and there was another steep climb through woodland and along a grass track. The climb was about three-quarters of a mile long. At one stage I was reduced to speed walking, the climb was that sheer. But waiting at the top of the hill were cheering crowds, hemming in the runners as they lined both sides of the path. The crowds were brilliant, shouting encouragement as the route to the finish bizarrely took runners through a shopping mall, and into the town square.

I was told the distance was three miles - my watch measured 2.8 miles, and a mark of how tough the climb was could be found that my watch read 21 minutes 19 seconds. Painfully slow! It was a lovely race set is wonderful countryside, and it felt fantastic to be part of a community event.

27. Neolithic Cani-Cross @ Stonehenge, Wiltshire.

THIS was a first - the first time I have ever run a race with a dog! The event was the Neolithic Cani-X, a four-mile run from the Bustard Inn on Salisbury Plain to Stonehenge.

It's a race which took a lot of advanced organisation, particularly as I don't have a dog. Fortunately, two friends who I met in March at a Hash on the Isle of Wight came to my rescue when Deanna and Rick kindly lent me their beautiful four-year-old Labrador, Boykie.

They came over to the mainland on Saturday afternoon and in the evening we had our first run together. Boykie wore a harness which was attached to a lead, which in turn was attached to a belt strung around my waist. We found some fields along by the River Hamble – Howard's Way country, with yachts and dinghies gracefully plying their way up and down the waterway in the early summer sunshine. For our first practice run, Boykie took off like a bat out of hell. It was hard to keep him under control and he had to be reined back. I had no control whatsoever. Boykie was full of energy who wanted to run and run and run.

Come race day, Rick, Deanna and myself drove to Stonehenge in Rick's van to meet all the other competitors and their dogs. Some of the owners had raced before; others were new to the game. Deanna stayed behind at

Stonehenge to enjoy a spot of sight-seeing as we were shepherded onto a coach and driven to the start. Several American tourists, passengers on the Queen Mary 2 who were wearing some extremely loud clothes, had just stepped off a coach which had driven up from Southampton to visit the stones. They looked on in amazement at the sight of these dogs being led up the steep coach steps and then taking their places in seats by the window. The video camera footage would have been great. "Hey, Hank. Take a look at these dogs. Ain't they cute?!!!" The coach did smell a bit with all these hounds on board.

Ours was the shorter race distance of four miles from Bustard Inn; some runners and their faithful friends had been ferried to Charlton Clumps for a 13-mile half marathon race to Stonehenge. Rick, Boykie and myself went to the pub for a nutritional pre-race bacon roll and coffee before getting ready for the race. It was deserted inside this aged pub, so we made the most of the moment before the start which was right next to a red-flagged military zone at the heart of Salisbury Plain. Huge muddy tank tracks, now hardened by a recent spell of warm weather, criss-crossed the path in front of us. We put ourselves near the front of the 31 other competitors knowing that Boykie would be off like a shot. And he was. He blasted off like a rocket, and I thought I was going to come a cropper as I hurdled the tracks and skated across the rough terrain before we got onto the firmer ground of the footpath. I was petrified because I had no control of Boykie. It was amazing I managed to stay on my feet.

Very quickly we lost Rick. We were going at close to six minute mile pace, and I was trying to rein in Boykie to a steady pace. In front of us there were two other runners as the route picked its way along paths by Salisbury Plain.

I had a funny feeling that we might even win this one. I had the stamina and the running in my legs. The game plan was to close in on the leaders as we edged towards the finish, and then unleash Boykie over the final half mile for a momentous victory with Deanna waiting for us at the finish line by Stonehenge.

We went through the half way point by the water station. Rick was way behind us, but Boykie was going well. And then, without warning, he stopped! Boykie cocked his leg and went for a wee. Once he'd had his constitutional, my four-legged friend began sniffing the grass, and simply wouldn't budge. "Come on Boykie, we can win this," I chided. I got out a water bottle, squirted it into his mouth and on his head, but Boykie was simply disinterested in running. Dogs! Bloody dogs! Never work with children or animals!!

Soon we were passed by a flurry of dogs and their owners. It was like a scene out of that classic 1970s cartoon, Wacky Races. We were Muttley and Dastardly who had seen their masterly plan blow up in their faces with the finishing line in sight. The dynamic duo were humiliated as Penelope Pitstop, the Boulder Mobile, the Creepy Coupe, Professor Pat Pending and not forgetting the Ant Hill Mob roared past to take the chequered flag! In reality the two leaders headed over the ridge as Boykie sniffed the flora and fauna nursing an "Am I bovvered?" type of attitude. All I wanted to do was to shout "MUTTLEY, do something!"

Rick soon caught up with us bemused by the lack of action. Boykie was tired and didn't want to run. We rested him, and then began walking a bit, before getting into a trot. Soon Boykie was running with us, though a little slower than before. We still caught a few runners and their dogs, and the familiar circle of stones at Stonehenge soon loomed into sight.

As we entered a field and the finishing straight, Boykie pricked up his ears, he could see Deanna and a photographer, and he started sprinting. What a poser! I was off in pursuit being dragged along with Rick alongside. We crossed the finish line in around 32 minutes for seventh place. Rick and I were handed a medal, but I gave mine to Boykie and put it around his shoulders. He looked well pleased with the medal draped around his neck. As for me and Rick, we were dog tired!

28. Penicuik 10k @ Penicuik, Midlothian, Scotland.

SIX races in seven days taking in 47.5 miles of some of the toughest terrain in the United Kingdom – this was going to be a tough schedule over one week in mid-May. My sponsors Flybe flew me to Scotland for my first foray north of the border during this runner year. Lying ahead was the arduous Cape Wrath Challenge in the far north of Scotland, but I was looking for a gentle warm-up race on the Saturday so stumbled upon the Penicuik event which seemed to fit the bill.

The flight from Southampton was unfortunately delayed, so this meant a quick dash from Edinburgh Airport to Penicuik, which lies 10 miles south of the Scottish capital. Runners changed in the High School which was a throw back to the days of Goodbye Mr Chips. It had a lovely rustic feel to it; one of those old-style gymnasiums with shiny wooden floors and climbing frames stationed around the sides of the walls.

One of the organisers, Susie Maxwell, was there to meet me. In the months leading up to the race we had corresponded by e-mail as she had followed my racing schedule closely. In the school canteen, which was to serve as race headquarters, Susie had posted up a flier with my photograph and details of the racing plan for the year. I also caught up with a sage of the Penicuik Harriers called George, who told me about the history of the area, how Penicuik was once a hive of industry with two paper mills and home to the Edinburgh Glass Company. Now that had all gone and Penicuik was now a sleepy suburb of Edinburgh. The biggest attraction is the local Ikea!

The weather was slightly overcast for the race which started beside a park, sending runners through the town centre and towards a stinker of a hill. "This isn't a hill, it's a Munro," I suggested to one of the runners who was breathlessly struggling up this steep, steep obstacle. The hill leading out of the town is a good half mile long, rising in two stages. At times you were almost running on the spot. I pushed on the best I could, trying to run within myself and then striding out on the summit.

I found myself running most of the way with a lady called Isobel Knox from the fantastically named Hunters Bog Trotters. They are a running club based in Edinburgh who sport a disgusting chocolate brown vest. Isobel was good company as we battled our way out of Penicuik, along the back lanes making our way through the back markers.

The beginning of the race may be tough, but the second half of the Penicuik 10km was a dream. It consisted of a spiralling downhill run for a good mile or two, twisting and turning along the road into town. With Isobel on my shoulder we pushed and paced hard. She was receiving plenty of support on the course which encouraged me to not lose the lady.

A couple of turns into the town, and a slight uphill before a final finish in the park with a 250 metre sprint. Isobel had tired a little by this stage, so I sprinted to the line for 70th place in 44 minutes 6 seconds, five seconds ahead of Isobel. We exchanged a few words at the end, she then hoisted a rucksack on her back and shouted "I'm off to work!"

It was a lovely race, and as seems to be the way with Irish and Scottish runs, there was a wonderful spread of sandwiches, cakes and tea laid on in the school hall afterwards. Here was a fantastic way to kick off my running week in Scotland.

29. Cape Wrath Challenge, Durness, Scotland – Loch Eriboll Half Marathon.

THERE can be few places in the British Isles where you can easily leave your front door unlocked, where you won't see one piece of graffiti daubed on a wall and where crime is virtually non-existent. Durness is the last stop in mainland UK. It is the most north-westerly inhabited place in mainland Britain, home to some 320 people; a collection of scattered townships and farms. Walk in a straight line from Durness and the next landfall is the North Pole! Yes, I know technically that the North Pole doesn't have any land since it is floating ice, but you get the cut of my jib!

Durness is as remote as remote can be, enjoying a leisurely pace of life far removed from the hustle and bustle of 21st century living. It is tucked in the top left-hand corner of Scotland, a tough two-hour drive from Inverness along roads which weave their way through the rugged mountains and barren moorland of the Highlands.

For one week every year, Durness hosts the Cape Wrath Challenge – five races in six days in May, culminating in a marathon which, with 2,500 feet of climb, is described as one of the toughest marathons in the UK.

Durness is a very close community. One of the town's characters is Ronnie Lansley who tells of the history of the area in his book "Durness Past and Present". Among the many interesting tales is one about the Durness body snatchers and the two men who removed a body from a grave at Balnakeil cemetery, setting off with the body in the back of the cart. They stopped on their way at the Durness Inn, leaving the cart parked in the corner. The two men slipped a nosebag on the horse to keep him quiet, and just in case anyone looked into the cart while they were away, they dressed the body in a cloak and hat, and propped it up in the driver's seat with a whip in its hand. While the body snatchers were inside the inn, a local lad walked by, gave the figure a poke and the body fell backwards off the seat.

After recovering from the fright, the boy realised what was happening, told a friend and they lifted the body out of the cart, hiding it close by. The boy then dressed himself in the cloak and hat, grabbed the whip in his hand and took the place of the corpse. The body imposters came out of the inn after a few drams, sat the body between them and set off home. The body imposter nudged one of the men and then the other. The two men quarrelled, and then fell silent as they noticed the corpse was getting warmer. The corpse turned to the men and looking them straight in the face in the moonlight, he said in a low voice: "Aye, and if you had been in hell as long as I have, you'd be feeling pretty warm yourself". The two men froze with fright, screamed and ran off into the night! The young fellow drove himself back to Durness, fetched the minister and reburied the body. No-one came to collect the horse and cart which was sold, and the money went towards the young man who bought a small croft where he settled.

In truth, here is a place where folk understand the true sense of community, working and pulling for each other. The remoteness of the area is its beauty. From Edinburgh, Liz and I drove to Durness via an overnight stop with my uncle who lives just outside of Perth. The final 70 miles from Inverness was along single-track roads which makes driving problematic and interesting. The jaw-dropping scenery anaesthetises the brain from the full-on concentration needed to traverse the narrow roads where when you see a crash barrier on a tight bend, it does mean - slow!

The countryside surrounding Durness is breathtaking; stunning cliff tops and empty beaches facing the Atlantic Ocean. Drive into the Highlands where you are greeted with valleys carved by glaciers millions of years before, shaped high and proud. Rocky hillsides on which sheep graze; moorland dappled with green, orange and browns. Nestled deep in the base of the valleys are still and peaceful lochs, inviting, but cold and deep.

On the Sunday evening, Liz and I checked into our very pleasant bed and breakfast before venturing to the village hall to meet the other runners. This was the fifth running of the Cape Wrath Challenge, and many were regulars delighted to be catching up with old friends. Runners had ventured from all parts of the kingdom to the north of Scotland – from Nottingham and East London, the Lake District and Kent, Merseyside and Cambridgeshire, as well as a fair sprinkling from Scotland. They were a pleasant, chatty lot, looking forward to the week with a mixture of excitement and apprehension. We were feeling unsure ourselves of what lay ahead.

Outside the village hall lies a surprising memorial to John Lennon. Who would have thought that the ex-Beatle would be revered in this part of Scotland? However, besides Durness Village Hall stands the John Lennon Memorial, a garden set out with a series of stones carrying lyrics from the song "In My Life". The connection is that John Lennon spent many of his holidays at the home of Bertie Sutherland, who married John's maternal aunt. He took Yoko Ono to this far flung corner of the UK where he was clearly touched by the no frills, back-to-basics environment.

Come Monday morning and the first day of the challenge, the weather was bright and light – the sun rises at 4.45am in this part of Scotland during the summer and sets around 10pm.The first race of the week was the Loch Eribol half marathon. We were driven by minibus 13 miles out of Durness along a lonely, single-track road circling the magnificent lake which was bordered on both sides by sloping hills, decorated with specks of orange gorse among the lush grassland.

There were 57 of us lined up on the desolate road in the middle of nowhere, and with the blast of a hooter we were off. The front runners were fast as from the start half a dozen of them hared away at breakneck speed down the hill. I felt very heavy in those early stages and the first couple of miles were hard. Whether it was Saturday's race in Edinburgh, or I was feeling generally lethargic it was difficult to know. I settled into a rhythm as we turned the lake to follow the road. A few vehicles passed us, their drivers honking horns and passengers waving encouragement. I found myself on my own for the entire way allowing me to take in the magnificent scenery - a rural green backdrop on my left, and the deepwater loch to my right.

Today, the loch is used for farming salmon, mussels and oysters, but it was once an historic naval anchorage. Loch Eribol was the last mainland port of call for HMS Hood before she was sunk by the German warship Bismark in 1941, and in 1945 the loch was used as a surrender point for the North Atlantic U-boats.

The weather was glorious for the start of the run alongside the crystal clear waters and under the watchful protection of the huge mountains of Cranstackie and Ben Spionnaidh. But an hour into the race there was a sudden five-minute hailstorm, whipped up by a piercing south-westerly wind, which stung the eyes with salt and numbed your face.

The hills were testing and searching. Towards the end of the race we were faced with one monstrous climb where the hill kicked in twice by a chicane. You craned your neck to see the runners ahead of you. The rise hurt the hamstrings, and scorched the lungs. A mile or two later, there was even a nasty little kick to the finish with a testing uphill stretch. I was being slowly caught by the first lady in the race, Zoe Woodward from Eton Manor AC in East London, and was determined to finish ahead of her as we reached the finish line at Durness Village Hall - a blue inflatable finish marker. I was pleased with my time of 1 hour 38 minutes 52 seconds, which was good going for the rugged countryside, and 19th overall.

30. Cape Wrath Challenge, Durness, Scotland – Sangomore Hill Run.

THE Sangomore Hill Run forms the second day of competition. It's a chance to change out of the road shoes and don trail wear for the 5.5 mile trek along some of the lower slopes of the hills around Durness. I wasn't feeling great and a little bit sickly. The half marathon the day before had been fine, and the legs were good. But my stomach felt decidedly dodgy, maybe the after-effects of the quiz the night before, so I treated this as a very gentle training run.

Runners set out on a beautiful morning along a muddy track towards Loch Caladil. We then climbed onto the moor to the edge of Loch Meadaidh and crossed a series of stepping stones by a ford at Alt Smoo Burn. Those who wanted to venture back on the shorter four-mile route could do so here. The rest of us started the ascent towards Beinn Ceannabeinne. This is an ancient track once used by villagers to drive cattle from Durness up onto the hill and the summer pastures. It was a tricky little climb, but once at the top, the view was splendid overlooking the sea and the village of Durness below.

We then had a one mile descent, a free-rolling run downhill towards the Smoo Cave, and a final stretch of road uphill to the finish at the village hall. My stomach didn't feel too smart, but this was a smooth run when, despite not putting in a lot of effort, I finished 24th. I ran part of the way with a genial Irishman called Patrick, who lives in Aberdeen and runs for the Aberdeen Metro club. He rediscovered the sport five years ago after a spell out of running. Patrick looks and sounds like a character out of the TV comedy, Father Ted, and as we ran through this wonderful countryside he said to me: "I thank God that I am able to run each day." Thank God, indeed.

31. Cape Wrath Challenge, Durness, Scotland – Round Durness Race

RACE three was the Round Durness Run; three races in three days. Of all the five races being staged in the remote outpost of Scotland, this event sounded like a doddle; an 8.4-mile saunter around the tracks and trails surrounding the pretty village.

Steve from the Warrington Road Runners and Gerard from Stroud & District AC in Gloucestershire, two old hands who were staying at the B&B with us, underplayed the difficulty of the terrain we were going to face when the race was discussed over a traditional Scottish breakfast. This was one of the hardest races of the week; challenging and unrelenting. After taking it easy the previous day, I was determined to go out hard for this Wednesday work-out.

We set out from the village hall, which sits on top of a hill just outside Durness, and headed down a track towards Loch Caladil, then out onto the A838 which leads out of the village. As we reached the crest of the hill the view was jaw-dropping. Set out in front of us was Loch Boralie and Keodale Pier, surrounded by mountains. It was an awesome.

I was going well, very well, working nicely with Zoe Woodward from Eton Manor AC, who I had just edged out in the half marathon on Monday. Zoe was to go on and win the individual ladies' prize from the week. But just as we turned off the road by the entrance to the ferry, so the hard work began. This was a slog over some steep hills and tricky terrain around the Durness Golf Club, down towards Balnakeil Beach and up to the headlands of Adonmhor and Sanateachal.

Loch Boralie and the plantation area, including the golf course, is a designated site of scientific interest. The area from the coast inland is an area rich in archaeology. At Aodann Mhor, there was a farming township until the early 17th century. This was swept away by the third Lord Reay, chief of the Clan Mackay, when he remodelled his lands at Balnakeil. Along the wall, separating the headland from the fields we could pick out the run rigs; long narrow cultivation strips, and on a small, precarious headland, the faint traces of a monastic cell could be seen.

The beauty of the area was somewhat lost by the gruelling second half of the run. The climbs were energy-sapping almost reducing you to a walk.

I was beginning to feel the start of a blister in my left foot which exercised the mind. By this time Zoe had forged ahead and I was left hanging on for as long as I could. We soon arrived back in Durness, through the village square and back to the hall, with a killer climb up a steep hill known as the Caa. The gradient is so severe it is hard to know what it measures. Certainly driving up the hill in a car, you need to ease down to second gear on a bend two-thirds up the hill. The finish line at the village hall was a blessing. I placed 17th for a good run, but nursing a bloody sore blister for my efforts.

The great thing about the Cape Wrath Challenge is that despite the competition, it is not over the top and intense. It is a race week organised by runners for runners. Folk are happy to talk about running without becoming too obsessive. Equally, the week is sprinkled with a host of social events - a quiz, walks, abseiling, boat trips, Scottish dancing. It is a wonderful environment to meet new people and to make friends. It is why runners travel from all over the country year after year for this annual pilgrimage to the far north coast of Scotland.

Among those I met was local photographer, Kevin Arrowsmith who, along with wife Frances, uprooted from their home on Teesside to set up in this remote outpost of the British Isles.

"Our first visit to Durness was in 2003 having read an article in Runner's World magazine about the Cape Wrath Challenges," recalled Kevin. "The description of the area and the running events convinced us to take an early holiday up there, camping with our two children. We had an amazing week. The running events were exceptional, the scenery stunning and the community spirit inspiring. We simply had to return again the following year."

And that they did. Their pilgrimages to Sutherland became an annual event where they developed new friendships with runners and locals. "It became a breathing space away from the hustle and bustle of urban life on industrial Teesside," added Kevin. "Re-adapting to life on Teesside after visiting Durness became a little more difficult each year. I had become disillusioned with corporate life in my own career and hoped for the opportunity to develop an alternative career in photography. So, when my wife realised that there was a vacancy for a community nurse/midwife, the dream of relocating to Durness suddenly seemed feasible."

Frances applied for the job, was offered the post and ever since the couple have been turning their wonderful dream into a reality. "The reality has more than fulfilled our expectations," said Kevin. "Community values are strong, things happen at an altogether more civilised pace and, most importantly, people have time for each other. Eight months in, we still have to pinch ourselves and remind each other that we live here. While faces and place names are becoming familiar, the beauty of this area never ceases to astound."

32. Cape Wrath Challenge, Durness, Scotland – Target Zero: Balnakeil to Faraid Head Beach Run.

TYPICAL of the laid back atmosphere of the week was Thursday's race known as the Target Zero: the Balnakeil to Faraid Head Beach Run. This race not only attracts competitors taking part in the week-long challenge, but runners from the village and dozens of schoolchildren get involved too. Many were kitted out in fancy dress. We had mermaids, Neptune, a ghost, plus runners kitted out in their nightclothes!

The run consists of a three mile saunter along the beach, through the dunes and back. Running without a watch, global positioning system, or any sort of ready reckoner, the idea is to get back to the finish by Balnakeil Church closest to your target time. Working on the basis of seven-and-a-half to eight minute mile pace, I had predicted a time of 23 and a half minutes for the fun run.

Water soon seeped into running shoes as we set out along the beach. Carrying a blister from the day previous didn't help matters. That didn't detract from a very pleasant run where I finished in just over 24 minutes and some 90 seconds outside of my time. Not bad, but way off the mark. One runner managed to finish within nine seconds of their target and another, incredibly, was spot on with 21 minutes exactly. Surely there should be a steward's enquiry!!

33. Cape Wrath Challenge, Durness, Scotland – Cape Wrath Marathon Relay.

THE finale to the Cape Wrath Challenge is the marathon itself on the Saturday. It is regarded as one of the most challenging 26-milers in the UK with more than 2,415 feet of climb over rugged hills.

Normally, the Cape Wrath Marathon begins from Keodale with an 11-mile run to the lighthouse by the Cape, and then a run back towards the ferry. The clock is stopped while a boat takes runners across the small stretch of water, before the final four-mile dash to Durness. I was sorely tempted to take part though Liz had reminded that I would owe her £100 if ever I entered another marathon after being so adamant about the prospect after London. However, besides the marathon there was also a series of two, three and five-person relays. Coming at the end of a hard week, I chose an 11-mile leg as part of a three-strong marathon relay which is organised on a time trial basis – the three times are then tallied for a finish.

However all the best laid plans of mice and men went to pot when we woke on the Saturday morning. It was blowing a fair old gale outside and there was no way we were going to be able to get on the ferry to cross for the marathon. For the first time in the race's history, the marathon would not reach to the lighthouse.

Instead the marathon runners set out against a fierce headwind from Durness on a 13-mile out and back run along a single track road which cut a swathe through the steep hills. For the 11-milers like myself, and those running the shorter four-mile legs, we were bussed out to a remote start and sent on our way.

Low cloud hung over the mountains, rain swept horizontally and fortunately, with a downhill start, the wind was right on our tails. We were flying for five miles and even with the rain lashing across our faces, this was the most exhilarating running I have ever done. The first mile marker I reached in 5 minutes 50 seconds, then just over 12 minutes for the second mile – I had never run this fast before. It was incredible. I felt light and airy. My legs, cooled by the rain, bounced off the asphalt, as my body was pushed forward by the wind. Even when I went to clear my throat, the phlegm sailed for yards!

Rain soaked through your clothes to the skin, but that didn't detract from the experience. Once again the scenery was astonishing despite the grey backdrop; fast-flowing streams, deep and dark lochs, steep rocky headlands. Throw in the spectacular mountain scenery, the wild countryside, and the solitude of silence with barely a vehicle on the road, and it made for perfect running.

The marathon runners who were battling against the headwind came towards us looking exhausted and dishevelled – and with a long, long haul ahead you couldn't help feel sorry for them. I had a glorious run. The rain soon passed and the sun shone. I maintained a good speed, which slowed only with one tough uphill stretch by the ferry. We then swung into Durness and headed towards the village hall faced with a severe headwind which reduced you to a crawl.

But once at the crest of the hill, I managed to catch some runners who I had given a four-mile start to and crossed the line in line in a time of 1 hour 18 minutes 1 second – which, for me, was quick. It brought the curtain down on a great week of racing, a superb run and a wonderful way of awakening the senses.

That evening at the prize-giving reception, I met Bruce Tulloh, now 71 and one of the great British middle distance runners, who had come to Cape Wrath especially to compete in the relay. Bruce was one of the finest runners of his generation winning the European 5,000m title in Belgrade in 1962. He competed in the 1960 Olympics in Rome and during an illustrious career he held the British two-mile, three-mile and six-mile UK records, as well as running under four minutes for the mile on those famous cinder tracks.

Bruce was famous for running barefoot on the track where he left others trailing. "I didn't always run barefoot," he recalled. "That depended on the track I was running on. However, bare foot felt more comfortable and the grip was good. Without a shoe you were much lighter in the stride and able to cover more ground. Even with the lighter shoes around today, if I was running on the track now I would probably go barefoot."

He added: "Running is basically a poor man's sport. To do well requires many hours of hard work a week, with a slim chance of success. If you have plenty of time and no money, as in Kenya, it's worth doing, but if you have to risk your career and your income it is not so attractive. If there are thousands of talented people training hard, as in Kenya, the standard goes up, but if you can win most of your races with a 30-minute 10km, the standard does not go up.

"I ran a record 27 minutes 23 seconds for six miles in 1966 – which is around 28min 23sec for a 10k, with half a dozen Brits right behind me. In the Sixties, a good runner had the reward of overseas trips, but nowadays you can have an overseas holiday for the price of a week's wage."

Since turning 65, Bruce tries to exercise 30 miles a week. "Some days I cycle instead and count 10 miles on mountain bike as five miles' running. I have always enjoyed running and will continue to do so until the day I die."

34. Mull of Kintyre Half Marathon

THE Argyll and the Kintyre Peninsula couldn't have been more different from the Highlands of Scotland which I had visited a week earlier.

Where in the far north I had found strikingly high mountains, grass and rocky slopes peppered with gorse and lavender, my new destination was all about tranquil glens, wooded hillsides, breathtaking bays and beaches.

The drive from Glasgow to Campbeltown, the main focal point on Kintyre, was slow but scenic. The road hugged the shoreline, heading up one isle and down the next, looking across lochs and then the open sea to the isles of Jura and Islay, and 12 miles distant across the Irish Sea, the mountains of Antrim in Northern Ireland where I had run just two months earlier.

I was in Campbeltown for the Mull of Kintyre Half Marathon. Only in its second year, the 13-miler had received plenty of positive reviews from its opening sortie, and though this meant a second trip to Scotland in consecutive weeks I felt this was a race which I could not miss. It describes itself as one of the most scenic half marathons in the UK and certainly lived up to its name with a wonderfully varied course down country lanes on the outskirts of Campbeltown, and even a brief stretch along the beach.

There can be no half marathon like it. A pipe band accompanied runners as they lined up for the start by the harbour where a fleet of half a dozen fishing smacks lay tethered. On the way to the start I spotted a flier pinned to a noticeboard with details of a sermon due to be given that morning by Kirsty-Anne Burroughs at the St Kiaran's Scottish Episcopal Church was entitled: "Long distance running and the Christian faith – are there connections?" That would have been interesting to hear as. I often need a prayer or two to get round the course.

The half marathon runs side by side with the 10km event and both races started together before splitting off after one mile. For the half marathon, the course was a gentle run out into the countryside, past the airport, and along the western coastline where the course headed over sand dunes and onto the beach. This was a first; a half marathon on a beach. The tide was kind, and though the surf rushed up to the edge of the course, there was no danger of getting wet on a 400 metre run up to a point and back. Last year, a lone piper played a lament to runners reaching the mark, but this year he had been given the Sunday off.

On the way back across the dunes, I crashed into one of the slower runners who was gingerly tracing a path between the clumps of grass and dunes. The track was wide enough for an articulated lorry, but this blob of running lard just couldn't get to grips with the sandy cambers. I bounced off this guy's stomach and onto my fat backside. "Sorry mate, couldn't move out of the way quick enough," he offered by way of apology. I've seen faster turning oil tankers!

The downhill run into Campbeltown was cruise control, lifted by wonderfully generous crowds who lined both sides of the road. For that final stretch I ran with a guy called Syd Gallacher, deputy headmaster of the local school and who I had met the night before at a race pasta party at the town's leisure centre. Syd had never run faster than 1 hour 40 minutes for a half marathon before. I told him to stick on my shoulder and he'd get a personal best guaranteed. We pushed on at a pace, easing into Campbeltown on a gentle downhill stretch to finish in 1 hour 35 minutes and 21st place.

Syd was delighted with the five-minute PB. He kindly offered me hospitality at his home afterwards with a chance to take some tea, get a shower and take part in a Ceilidh at the Victoria Hall in Campbeltown that evening, featuring the World and European Championship-winning Kintyre Schools Pipe Band. But I had to decline as I shot back to Edinburgh airport to catch a plane back to Southampton - a 180-mile drive to the Scottish capital along the tight Kintyre roads, which took almost four hours.

35. Beat the Baton @ Battersea Park, London.

THE reason for heading back south so quickly was because I had a race on the Bank Holiday Monday in London's Battersea Park for a race called Beat the Baton. This was a run which I had read about a year earlier which took part in Huntingdon and was organised by the charity Sue Ryder Care – the race consisted a couple of laps on a 5km course accompanied by the Royal Philharmonic Orchestra belting out a string of classics.

Twelve months on and the friendly folk at Sue Ryder Care must have felt their hearts sink when they saw the weather forecast. It was awful. The drive up the A3 to London's Battersea Park was marked by the windscreen wipers clearing heavy rain as dark, menacing clouds hung overhead. It was such a shame because Beat the Baton deserved picnic conditions. Instead, it got batten down the hatches weather.

Despite the rain, wind and a severe drop in temperature to 7c, hundreds of runners and joggers braved the conditions, many wearing the yellow Sue Ryder plastic covers to protect themselves in the warm-up for the race. A huge stage had been set up for the Royal Philharmonic Orchestra to play on, and massive television screens stood by the side. There were also food stalls and tents.

We really should have been picnicking in the park with the children and enjoying the green surroundings of central London, with the familiar towers of Battersea Power Station, made famous by the front cover of Pink Floyd's 'Animals' album, looming large. Instead, we were forced to eat our picnic in a car, and then wrap up as if it was mid-January before dashing to the start. Still, it was funny how the traffic wardens were doing brisk business in the park.

Liz, and my three boys Micah, Leo and Ross joined me for the race. Micah and Leo were on supporting and photographic duties, and despite the miserable weather they were brilliant. Liz agreed to run the race, and for the first time in the challenge Ross took part. A few days earlier I had taken delivery of a specially-made running stroller for Ross. Despite his severe autism, Ross can walk. He likes to run in short spurts, but would never be able to bound his way to 5km. The stroller is designed and built by the Hampshire-based company, Delichon Limited. It doesn't come cheap, but for Ross it meant he could participate in this year-long adventure. The buggy is a nifty piece of engineering, lightweight and easy to assemble, which will give my son mobility and security even in his teenage years.

Ross was strapped in to the buggy, and wrapped up like a North Sea fisherman. The hooter went off and the Royal Philharmonic struck up the familiar strains of Rossini's William Tell Overture as we pressed on around the puddle-strewn paths of Battersea Park.

It was raining and it was cold. The buggy was lightweight and easy to steer, even with Ross inside. Ross seemed unmoved by the experience, yet we were getting plenty of cheers from the spectators. Other runners were pointing us to their partners marvelling at the sight of this mad runner easing past them with a boy in his stroller. It was noticeable, though, how towards the end of the run how those being overtaken were less than happy at being passed by Ross and his dad! It was as if we were making fun of them by cruising past in a buggy.

We kept pace with Liz, but in truth Ross and I could have gone faster. This wasn't a race, more of a fun run, but I wonder what time we could have achieved for 5 kilometres if we had gone hell for leather. We wouldn't have won, but the standard of runners was so mixed - most were joggers and occasional runners - that I think we could have made a top 10.

It was nice to hold back and to enjoy the run, as the Royal Philharmonic ran through a repertoire of classics; Orpheus in the Underworld, Vivaldi's Four Seasons, the 1812 Overture. We passed the bandstand for the second time to big cheers from the crowd close to the finish line and crossed in 25 minutes 30 seconds.

It was a fun experience. The experiment with running with a buggy had worked well. It hurt a little on the back, but that pain would ease with experience. Ross didn't seem at all perturbed, which was a relief. It was just a shame about the weather which, if it had been kinder, would have made a good day just brilliant.

"People don't know why we run, but it's the hard work you put into practice, and the reward you get from the race."

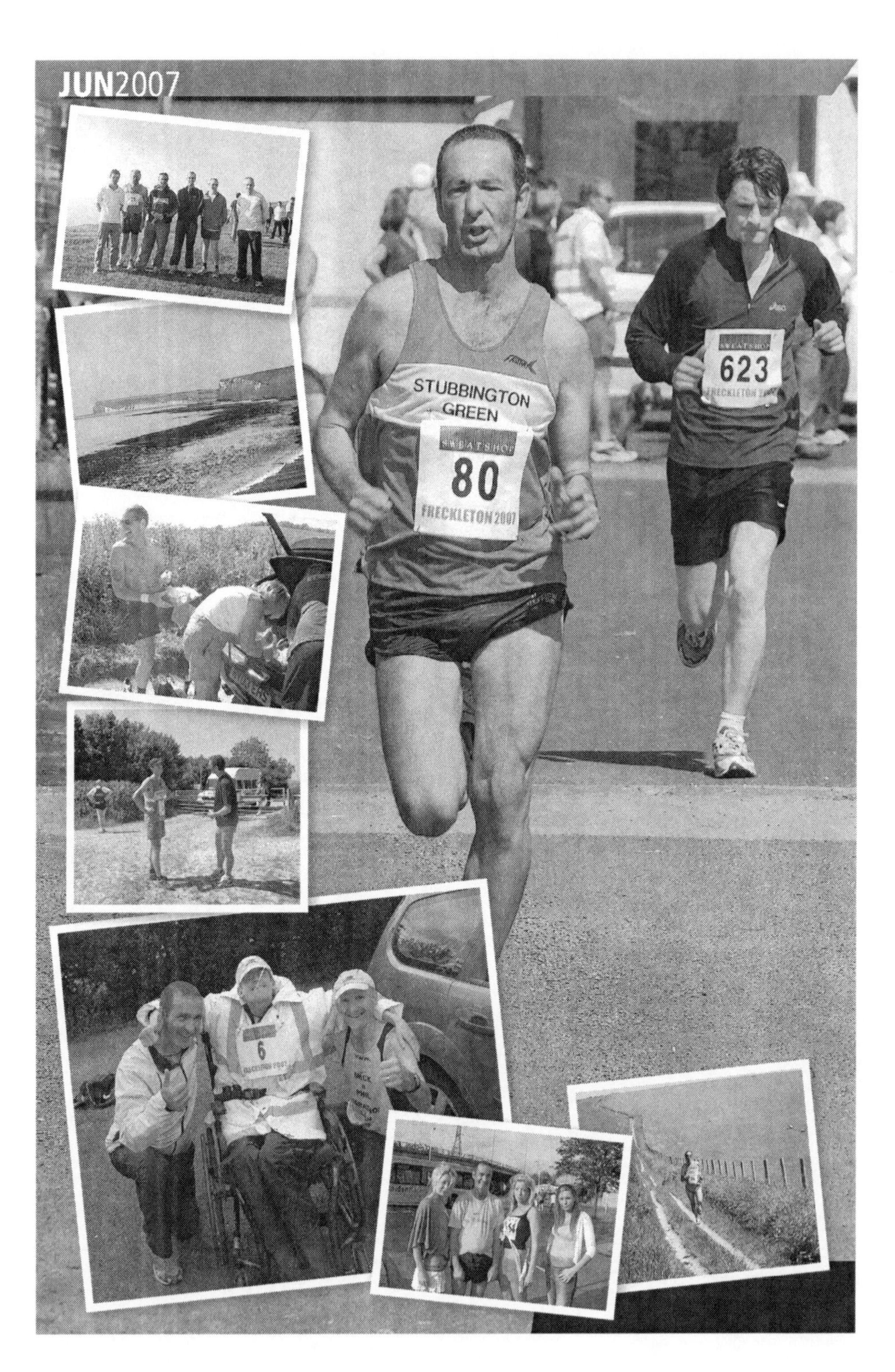
JUN2007
STUBBINGTON
GREEN
SWEATSHOP
80
FRECKLETON 2007
SWEATSHOP
623
6

JUNE

36. South Downs Way Relay – Beachy Head, East Sussex to Chilcomb, Hampshire.

RUNNING is full of pitfalls and hazards. For example, there are those numbskull motorists who as soon as they spot you crossing a road they're turning into, will put their pedal to the metal to re-enforce the message over who has the right of way.

Then there are the erratic pavement cyclists who seem determined to mow you down, and very occasionally you will meet those chronically-slow OAP scooters whose drivers like to perform the "left-right-left-right" dance as they meet you along narrow tree-lined avenues. Of course a low-hanging bus shelter roof, overnight pavement works, and in the countryside sudden rabbit holes or fallen trees which have scythed across a footpath, all make for interesting navigation.

And then there are animals. Come the glorious day of the revolution, as Citizen Smith once put it, let moronic and selfish dog owners be the first to face the Imperial firing squad. "Oh, he's only having fun with you," will be the plaintive cry from Dumb owner as Dumber dog is trying to take a bite out of your ankle. The owners think it is funny believing it as a comic diversion from their morning walk. For me, it's a pain in the butt, and any mutt who comes my way while I'm out running, cutting across my path or sniffing around the Asics Nimbus, gets a size 10 placed right across its derriere. At least with dogs you can anticipate whether trouble is coming, but cows? Not on your nelly!

This was the South Downs Relay on a blistering hot first Saturday in June. The event is probably harder than running a marathon. Spread over a single day, 47 six-strong teams set out from Beachy Head in East Sussex to Chilcomb near Winchester tracing the route of the South Downs Way on a 100-mile, 18 leg race. It is a gruelling, stamina-sapping event with each runner completing up to 18 miles over some testing ground.

Twelve months earlier, running for Stubbington Green Runners' B team, we unexpectedly finished second in our category. This year, the cow incident creamed our dreams of milking success for a second year running, despite feeling rather bullish about our chances on the morning of the race.

The drama unfolded near Firle Beacon, an 800 foot hill halfway between Eastbourne and Lewes on the first of my three legs. Running across the South Downs, the English Channel glistened and the Dieppe-bound ferry eased its way slowly towards France from Newhaven. Ahead of me on a gentle downhill stretch was a gate where milling about were a herd of cows heading towards a feeding trough cutting across a well-trampled path. Once the herd saw this dribbling vision in green hurtling their way, most of the cud-chewing crowd scarpered…except for one. The Victoria Meldrew of the bunch looked in my direction, stopped, and then just as I moved in front of the moody old cow to get out of her way (there's a moral to this story), Ermintrude kept going to her breakfast feast and we collided. I caught the cow squarely on the nose with my hip. Instinctively and stupidly, I turned round without breaking stride and apologised to the unfortunate victim of the assault; like she was going to answer back and say: "No worries, good luck." I did ask one of the other cows if I was going in the right direction, but she replied: "You need to go the udder way"!

The weather was boiling hot. Hours earlier, when we had set out from Beachy Head at seven o' clock it had been a beautiful crisp morning. It was the calm before the storm, a comforting breeze before a cloudless scorcher. Picturesque the South Downs may be, but the hills and some of the terrain is draining. Compound that with June temperatures which were in the 70s, and the South Downs Way relay is definitely not a race for wimps.

Some teams suffered badly. One runner was badly injured and the squad had to pull out, another's vehicle broke down so they had to borrow a National Trust pick-up to complete the journey. But our day went down the pan after one of our team, Eric, twisted his ankle after putting his foot down a rabbit hole, and somewhere between the pain and distraction our man later lost his way. A seven-mile run which should have taken well under an hour took more than an hour and a half. Fortunately, Eric was okay and with his foot heavily strapped thanks to Liz's first aid skills, he managed to complete the remaining two legs.

It was a hell of a day. Our team of six runners plus two drivers, one of whom was Liz, had set out in two cars from Southampton at 5am to get to Beachy Head for our early start. We'd worked out the logistics of the race with a precision which Gulf War commanders would have been proud of; the two team cars leapfrogging each other at the starts and finishes of each leg, runners changing cars, while food, drinks plus changes of clothing were stashed in the car boots. Move over General Schwarzkopf, we had it sussed. If only our military planning matched our running and navigational skills.

From a racing point of view, we were badly behind. Any chances of winning a medal had been blown early on, but that didn't matter. As a team of six, we were all closely matched in terms of ability - middle-pack runners capable of completing 10km between 40 minutes and 45 minutes. We were here to compete safely and enjoy the relay, without the expectation of winning anything.

My next leg began at Saddlescombe, just north of Brighton near Devil's Dyke. It was midday and the heat was searing. The climb to the top of the Dyke, another 700ft hill, was crippling. I'd had three hours' rest from my last run, and my muscles ached. The opening gambit is a climb which goes up and up and up. Progress is slow and painful before the path evens out. The saucily-named Fulking Hill, which makes you want to swear on the climb, Perching Hill and Edburton Hill followed in rapid succession before Truleigh Hill, at 216 metres or 708 feet hits you between the eyes. It was Truleigh horrible.

One of my Stubbington team-mates, Richard Thomas, who was running for the A team which was to finish second, ate up the hill like it was no obstacle at all. I plodded up it, swerving slowly past walkers and cyclists who rode in the opposite direction downhill. Truleigh Hill was the final test on leg 7, and a nice downhill finish towards a changeover point on the A283 at Upper Beeding, next to the River Adur.

I hopped into the support car with Liz to take on the map-reading role as we weaved our way around the West Sussex countryside to each of the stop off points. As a team we were running well, but losing those 40 minutes early on was critical and we found ourselves at the back of the pack.

By the time of the leg 13, my final leg, there were only a couple of teams behind us. We had no-one to chase. I was dreading this last leg, the longest and toughest of them all - and regarded as one of the hardest on the South Downs. The start is by the A286 near Cocking north of Chichester, and finishes at Harting Hill in Hampshire, just a stone's throw from Petersfield. You're tired for starters. You've been on the go for almost 12 hours, your legs are starting to seize them up and need an electric charge to get them jump started. The first 1.2 miles of this leg is a slow, uphill drag up a farm track. That is the appetiser. You climb to Linch Ball, Didling Hill and then Treyford Hill before flinging a sharp right by the Devil's Jumps. When I checked out this route 12 months ago, I missed the turn totally and ended up half a mile down the path by a pub. Several runners that day made the same mistake.

Because of my busy race schedule this year, I'd not had a chance to recce any of my legs and this one concerned me most. For the Sussex section of the South Downs Way, the tracks are well marked and the way is pretty obvious. But once you get into Hampshire, the signposting goes awry and at the Devil's Jumps crossroads, there is no marking for the South Downs Way. I was struggling by this time, not only through tiredness but with a severe stitch which was cramping my running. My chest was sore and I had no rhythm at all. I wanted to stop, and had this not been a team race I would have. Instead I pressed on knowing the horror which awaited.

Half way into the 6.5 mile leg you hit Pen Hill which is sheer and severe; the only way is up a grassy trail. At the top, there is light relief, for the downhill, but in front lies Beacon Hill which stands at 800 feet tall. The climb is 164 feet. Only 164 feet, but the gradient is so sharp, and the path so rocky that even with a good run at the hill it is virtually impossible to run up. You have to speed walk.

At the summit, an equally sharp downhill greeted you to Bramshott Bottom, followed by an assault up chalky Harting Down, and then a fifth and final energy-sapping climb towards the car park.

Liz was waiting at the top, cheering me on, with a camera clicking away. I ran past a couple having a barbecue and the food smelled great. My chest hurt, my legs were screaming - this was worse than the London Marathon. At least with the capital caper you run 26 miles in one go over relatively flat terrain. Here, you were running 18 miles in three spurts over more than 12 hours across very hilly and testing territory. Exhausted, I finished the leg in just under an hour, relieved the ordeal was over

There wasn't much time to rest, it was straight into the support car to catch up with the other runners.

Word had reached us that organisers were looking at a cut-off time for 7pm by the start of leg 16 at the gloriously named Sustainability Centre near Winchester. Any team which failed to reach this point by the benchmark time would be out. I couldn't believe the organisers would do this. Even though we still had 17.5-miles to go to the finish and with darkness falling in another 90 minutes, I persuaded organisers to give us another quarter of an hour. They gave us that 15 minutes, but it was nearly 7.30pm by the time our runner handed over the baton. Sod it, we were going to continue even though with dusk falling the organisers were removing the marshals and told us we could continue at our own risk. There was no way we were going to abandon a day's running. A couple of other teams behind us had been forced to give up and call it quits.

By the time Nick, our anchor leg runner, arrived at the finish at Chilcomb, the presentations were winding up, the barbecue had long since been eaten, it was virtually pitch black. It was 9.45pm, so we gathered round the inflatable finish tunnel to cheer Nick in. We finished the South Downs Relay in a time of 14 hours 15 minutes and 45 seconds. We didn't win anything, we didn't even get a sausage from the barbecue, but we gutsed it out and we finished - and that is what running is all about.

37. The Blaydon Races- Newcastle, Tyne & Wear.

WEEL, heor wu gan agyen reet inta Blaydon Toon for the Blaydon Races. Yep, the official anthem of the Geordie nation is celebrated every ninth of June when 4,000 runners gather in the centre of Newcastle for a 5.7-mile run to the town of Blaydon, just the other side of the River Tyne in the borough of Gateshead.

We need to go back to the 19th century to trace the origins of the Blaydon Races, which was originally a Victorian Music Hall song written by a Gateshead lad by the name of Geordie Ridley. It traces a coach journey from Newcastle to Blaydon. The first public performance of the song by Ridley was made on June 5th, 1862 as a testimonial for the Tyneside sporting hero, Harry Clasper. It was sung at Balmbra's Music Hall in Newcastle.

In 1862, the Blaydon Races should have been held on an island in the middle of the River Tyne at Blaydon, but they were called off when a heavy storm made it impossible for the horses to get to the race course. The storm is recorded in the last verse of the Blaydon Races, but most of the events referred to in the song took place in 1861. The last Blaydon Races were held in 1916, but were abandoned when a riot broke out following the disqualification of a winning horse.

Fast forward to the 20th century and the Nike Blaydon Race. The running race was the inspiration of Dr James Dewar of Blaydon Harriers who organised the first 24 races from 1981. Jim died in June 2004, just two days after the staging of the 24th event. Today, the Blaydon Race is a running event with an enormous amount of fanfare, including live music, can-can girls, the crowning of a Blaydon Belle, a pre-race rendition by runners of the anthem, before the Lord Mayor of Newcastle rings a handbell to herald the six o'clock start.

Runners start from outside the Balmbras pub making their way along the Scotswood Road, over the Scotswood Bridge which crosses the River Tyne and to the finish in Blaydon itself. Come Saturday evening, you could see the bemusement among the sprinkling of hen and stag parties in Newcastle City Centre about to embark on a long night of partying treated to the sight of thousands of runners milling around the streets limbering up in their party costumes.

I headed straight to Blaydon to park up before catching a bus ferrying runners to Newcastle. Blaydon is a huge disappointment. What a dump. Is it twinned with Chernobyl? The town is a dive featuring a soulless shopping centre stuck next to a bus station and the McDonald's. The only mention of the Blaydon Races I could find was a plaque fitted onto a wall of the shopping centre. With Blaydon, you're expecting a town steeped in history, rich in culture, celebrating such a glorious past, yet Blaydon is a town sadly in decay.

I couldn't wait to get out of the town and onto one of the buses which ferried runners into Newcastle itself. The difference couldn't have been starker. There I latched on to a couple of runners, Ken and Carol, who live in Sunderland and who at the weekend work as stewards at the Stadium of Light, home of Sunderland Football Club. They gave me a guided tour of this impressive and vibrant city. Newcastle was buzzing. The architecture is wonderful, the city centre perched on a hill overlooking the town was filled with shoppers enjoying the June sunshine, folk sat on the Grey memorial, others watching a trumpet-playing busker and all around them a growing number of runners ready for the race.

It was choca-bloc at the start. Some slower runners had crept to the front, and inevitably it was slow progress for the first mile as we wound our way out of the city. Ken and Carol had warned me the route wasn't scenic or inspiring, and they were right. It was spectacularly dull. Even though it was just after 6pm, conditions weree still hot and humid.

We crossed the Scotswood Bridge, the course then took a twisty run-in to Blaydon, past McDonald's up the hill, and then a sweep into the shopping centre car park. Everyone who finished came away with a pretty impressive goody bag which included a t-shirt, a bottle of beer, various snacks, plus a pease pudding and ham bap! I was so hungry, that I ate all the food on the drive down the A1 afterwards.

To make my day, as I was leaving to drive south I spotted the Blaydon Belle, the beauty queen chosen for the race. Nineteen-year-old Claire had just finished the run herself, was pretty flushed, pretty flustered and pretty. After a little persuasion, Claire and friends posed for photographs - purely for publicity purposes, you understand!

38. Asics Potters Arf @ Stoke-on-Trent, Staffordshire.

ONE of the perks of the year-long journey has been to visit parts of the British Isles I've not been to before. Ordinarily I wouldn't dream of holidaying in the far north-west of Scotland; give me a beach, warm sunshine and a good book – plus hot and cold running maids, and I'm like a pig in mud. This has been a wonderful opportunity to visit some incredibly scenic and spectacular places, to understand how dramatic and ever-changing is the landscape of our fair isles.

The flip side of the coin is that the journey has also taken in some places which would not win any tourism awards for beauty. Two that spring to mind are Blaydon and then Stoke-on-Trent which, by dint of an amazing coincidence of scheduling, was where I headed next during one visually-polluting weekend.

I've never particularly liked the Potteries. The area is grotty and in dire need of a lick of paint, and as for some of the women, well, put bluntly, you struggled to find a half decent looking lass at times. Seriously, try it! Take the test!!

I drove straight to Stoke from Newcastle on the Saturday evening, a 190-mile jaunt arriving at my hotel quite late. It was a bit of a ropey establishment which had seen better days, but I couldn't complain since the chef went out of his way to conjure up a late night steak and chips for me just as he was about to wend his way home. A shop alarm from a nearby store also kept me awake for most of the night, and what with feeling pretty tired and achey from the race in Blaydon, I wasn't looking forward to a half marathon in Staffordshire.

The race is based in Stoke-on-Trent city centre, or Hanley (I couldn't really get my head around what the difference is). Anyway, the place must have a triangle twinning link with Blaydon and Chernobyl. It's bigger than its Geordie rival, but the town looks like the set for BBC TV's Ashes to Ashes where rough and ready detective Gene Hunt would turn up any moment in his Ford Cortina. Stoke is nothing more than a 1970s shopping centre, and the surrounding area is lifeless. Some of the shops and homes look as though they haven't seen a lick of paint this century. The brickwork is brown and dirty, dotted along the race route were a couple of buildings which were merely derelict shells.

At one time there used to be a Potteries Marathon, but now it has been replaced with this tough half marathon which attracted a good-sized entry of about 1,000 runners. Listening to the race announcer chatting to the runners beforehand, organisers would like to see the entry field quadruple in size to become a leading race in the country.

Anyone who does enter should be warned. This race is hilly, very hilly! The shopping centre in Hanley sits on top of a hill, and during the race there were three very stiff climbs - including one at three miles which is a mile-long ascent, and then a stinker of a climb up Milton Road a couple of miles from the finish which leaves a lot of runners walking.

I was aching following Blaydon and after a couple of miles I nursed serious doubts whether, for the first time this year, I would make the distance. I felt drained of energy, and the knowledge of the big climbs was morale-sapping. Fortunately I started off slowly, very slowly, and that tactic worked in my favour. It allowed me to work my way through the field, picking off runners. I am a good hill runner, even though I hate them, so with the mile-long hill I overtook a good 25 runners.

On one of the earlier hills I was soon joined by Stewart, who lives nearby in Leek. He had run the race a few times but admitted he wasn't fit, and he stuck with me. Stewart's story was an interesting one. Six years ago he was a smoker - 20 a day - his marriage was doing down the pan, and his parents were not well. He faced a big life crisis, and decided to give running a go. He gave up the cigarettes, moved on with his relationship, and found through running that his life was all the better for it. "People were coming up to me a few months after I'd taken up running to say how well I looked," he said. "That felt good, and gave me the incentive to stick at it."

It was good to have Stewart's company because the miles ticked by easily. I left him at the final hill at Milton Road. I have one pace going up hills. I treat them like stairs, and I couldn't slow for Stewart.

The crowds were magnificent. Many had set up their own impromptu water stations. For once the route started and finished in the city centre - I lamented earlier this year how races in Stratford and York where it would have been wonderful to run through the city, had chosen a countryside course. There was no countryside running in Stoke, it was all urban hills and a shopping centre.

My time was slow, very slow. One hour 41 minutes, but I was glad to have finished. Another nice goodie bag to add to one from Blaydon, including a smart t-shirt and a Potteries plate.

39. Freckleton Half @ Freckleton, Lancashire.

IN the six months I've been racing around the British Isles, the one common question I'm asked at events, besides "Are you out of your tiny mind driving so far for each race?" is "Have you met Mick and Phil, the marathon lads?" From Scotland to Cornwall, it seems everyone in the running world knows Mick and Phil.

Our paths have crossed five times this year – in Watford, Stratford-upon-Avon, Dudley Kingswinford, in Stoke, and then a week later in Lancashire for the Freckleton Half Marathon. Theirs is an inspiring story and a testament to one man's absolute devotion to his son and who at the beginning of 2008 picked up the Jane Tomlinson Inspiration Award from Runner's World.

Mick Curry, 49, is an experienced runner, but his disciplined pattern of leisurely Sunday runs all changed with the birth of his son Phil, who suffers from cerebral palsy and a condition known as sodium valproate syndrome, which was the result of a difficult birth. Phil is a lovely young man but is totally dependent on those around him. He has no speech, limited mobility and every day has been a challenge for Mick and his wife, Dawn, who herself suffers from poor health.

"Nursing Phil through the years has driven my wife and me to mental breakdowns," said Mick who explained how in 2002 he was faced with an ultimatum from his wife – either take Phil running with you in his wheelchair, or pack it in because she could not cope with it any longer.

"I thought it was the end of things," said Mick. "For starters, would the wheelchair stand up to it, would Phil like it, and, most importantly, could I do this while pushing him? Running is hard enough at times, no matter what standard you are. This was make or break, all or nothing.

"We started with a two-mile fun run which took 17 minutes 45 seconds. We then moved to 10km which took 46 minutes and then tackled a ten-miler in a time of 1 hour 48 minutes. The final test was the full marathon where we achieved a time of 4 hours 12 minutes. This was fantastic. We were both loving it and, quite simply, we were having the time of our lives. The rest, as they say, is history."

Mick was telling me his tale in sun-kissed Lancashire for the oldest half marathon in the UK where the dynamic duo from Stratford-upon-Avon were taking part in their 137th 13-miler and their 238th race together. When their previous wheelchair broke at a race in Milton Keynes, fellow runners rallied round to buy the boys a new one having raised an amazing £5,500 within a month. That demonstrates just how much esteem they are held in within the closely-knit running community.

During our chat before the race, several well-wishers came up to wish the lads good luck and to share a conversation. They finished in a time of 1 hour 59 minutes and 43 seconds which was pretty good considering the sweltering conditions.

Finishing just ahead of them was the great Ron Hill, now aged 69, and the greatest runner of his generation, who clocked 1:53.10. Ron won the first Freckleton Half back in 1969 when he walked away with a set of ladders for his pains, and he still holds the course record of 1:04.45.

The Freckleton Half is a great race with its rolling lanes and countryside acting as a wonderful backdrop. The town is situated between Preston and Blackpool. I had a storming four-hour drive to Lancashire. When I settled down for a Sunday morning cup of tea and bacon buttie in Lytham St Anne's overlooking the Irish Sea, the weather was gorgeous.

It is the UK's oldest half marathon and one which is highly respected. It's no surprise. Race director Brian Porter and Wesham Road Runners have got this race booted and suited to a T. It is probably the best organised race around. On a very hot afternoon, Brian had set up five water stations offering both water and sponges, two shower stops, and copious marshals dotted around the course.

The warmth among the crowd was genuine. Hundreds lined the route, stood outside pubs with beers in hand, children on the side of the road cheered hoping to high-five, and residents sat in deckchairs encouraging everyone who passed, exchanging good-natured banter.

The race is part of a day of activities in Freckleton. The village is coated in bunting, there's a huge fun fair, and several side stalls line the main field, along with a steady commentary to generate a lively but friendly atmosphere. The one downside was the 2pm start. I hate afternoon starts. It puts the whole body clock out, such as what to eat at lunchtime. You are also running at a time of the day when the air is no longer fresh, when the humidity is intense.

Starting in Freckleton village, the route rolled out past the Birley Arms (one of five pubs en route) before reaching Lytham and some of the most scenic countryside on the Fylde coast. I started off steadily, and was rewarded with one of my best runs. My finish time wasn't my fastest by a long measure – 1 hour 38 minutes - but I just kept picking off runners one by one. I was only passed by two people throughout the 13 miles, but this was a very satisfying run since I was continually working between the packs and moving on. I didn't want the race to stop.

When I arrived at the finish, the race announcer, Andy O'Sullivan, was kind enough to mention my challenge as I moved through the finish funnel, and I received some warm applause and kind comments from those around. Organiser Brian Porter had given me the race number 80 in honour of the 80 races I was running, and with the race memento, which was a race mug, the motto "running is a mug's game" was inscribed.

A top race and a top bunch of people.

40. Humber Bridge Half Marathon @ Hull, Humberside.

I WAS unbelievably lucky with the running weather in June, from stifling heat on the South Downs Way to sultry running conditions in Lancashire. But in truth many were asking at this time: summer, what summer? For most of June and into July, the sun decided to pack its bags and go on vacation as the heavens opened continuously. This caused widespread flooding, initially in northern England and the following month in the west country. It was a miserable summer, lives were lost, properties destroyed and no-one even bothered to mention the hosepipe ban.

One of the worst hit places was Hull. The day before the big floods I visited the East Riding to compete in the Humber Bridge Half Marathon. The race weather was muddled; a mixture of cloudy skies, sunshine and towards the end of the race, light showers. Those showers were to turn heavier later in the day when towns such as Beverley, where Liz and I had stayed the night before with her family, and parts of Hull were flooded.

Later that week in Hessel, where the race started, one man drowned when he was swept into a drain he was clearing out. Television pictures of the flooding, the work of the rescue services and the devastating impact the floods were having on the lives of people made harrowing viewing. This was not Bangladesh but Yorkshire, and the impact was numbing.

I had travelled to Hull by train. It made a pleasurable diversion from sitting in the car for hours on end, trying to get a decent reception on the radio. The year of racing was the easy part, if only I could have been magically transported via a Bedknobs & Broomsticks bed to each venue, the task would have been so much easier. I don't particularly enjoy driving and my clapped-out BMW, a dirt-trap on wheels with sweet wrappers, Mr Kipling Bakewell tarts and drinks bottles lining the back of the car, along with errant bits of sports clothing, was getting beaten up with the miles.

By the end of the year I was to cover 20,000 miles around the British Isles through a combination of rail, plane and car. Given the choice I would have gone everywhere by either plane or train, just to have the chance to read and relax.

On the 18.30 from Kings Cross to Doncaster I found myself hemmed in by a very entertaining crowd of passengers in the seats around me, who were baiting the heavily-built and stern-faced female ticket collector, who looked like an extra out of Prisoner Cell Block H. Picking our way through a mountain of topics, these strangers in carriage D, generally put the worlds to right and so the journey passed quickly!

Picking events to run for this year-long schedule was not easy. In fact, the project started back in the summer of 2005; and even half way through the campaign I was still tinkering with the plan of 80 races as new ones appeared on the horizon. Top of the list were races that were interesting. There has to be some sort of focal point for taking part. There was no point, after all, of competing in eighty 10km road races trudging around an anonymous industrial estate. I was looking for races of character, runs with a bit of history, with something unusual about them. Geographically, I was keen to make sure these were spread throughout the UK. It would be so easy to choose 80 races within an hour's drive. Boy, would that have been cheaper!

The Humber Half Marathon was a race which appeared quite late in the schedule. For one, I was lacking a race in that part of the world, but this race appealed simply because here was an event based solely around a huge suspension bridge. The race attracted a couple of thousand runners. It was also part of the UK Inter Counties Half Marathon Championships, so the field was very competitive.

However the start was chaotic. From the parking arrangements on a muddy, straw-strewn field where the Air Cadets, who were directing cars, had no idea what was going on, to the start area itself which was not clearly defined, as runners hung around a waiting area until the appointed hour, it was a mess.

Once the race got going then everything settled down. I had been joined at the start by a lovely lady called Kerry, whose husband and two-year-old daughter waved her off from the start. A real bobby-dazzler, this was Kerry's first half marathon, coming off the back of running 46 minutes for the Humber Bridge 10km. Despite the obvious attraction of running with Kerry, I didn't think I would be seeing much of her after the start. But fair play, she had an amazing run and we ended up running the race together.

After the success the previous week of Freckleton, when I had started the half marathon sedately and then worked my way through the field, I had decided on a similar approach at the Humber Half with Kerry close by.

When the time came to step up the pace, it was clear Kerry was working hard, but would she be able to sustain the pace? I wondered whether to push on and really race this, or run with the lady in red beside me in her first ever half marathon? I wisely chose the latter option and it was the right decision. I had a really good run, probably among the most enjoyable run of the 40 races so far. It was eight minute mile pace throughout, nice and steady.

The half marathon route consisted of a couple of early loops before setting out across the Humber Bridge which is 2.2 kilometres long and stands 100ft high over the sludgy brown River Humber below. The weather was perfect, bright and sunny without being too hot. Running at a slower pace meant I could savour the views and enjoy the race. It was the first time I had run this way all year.

Kerry battled her way through. There were a couple of tough hills along the route, and she stuck at it. "Talk to me, Dave, talk to me," she called a couple of times as we slogged up one of the hills. Clearly distraction therapy was the key. One lady passed us up this belter of a climb at mile 9 and said to Kerry "you're looking so comfortable and cool - go on, show these guys how to race!"

We kept the pace steady, and towards the end began reeling in the runners. We had this one guy constantly in our sights; shaped like a weeble-wobble who was wearing a garish green vest along with grey and red skin-tight leggings. It was unsightly to look at and dispiriting to run behind. "We can't let the Weeble beat us," I said to Kerry. She smiled behind a grimace and cracked on.

As we strode over the Humber Bridge for a second time, this plucky young lady found a second wind and started to motor. "I want to run 1 hour 45 minutes," she pleaded. "Well, come on then, let's do it," I replied.

We passed the Weeble two or three times in a cat and mouse game; as soon as we rounded his shapely body to pass, he sped up to overtake. To be fair, the vision in lycra wobbled his way past one too many times and was to finish a few seconds in front of us. With a sprint at the end, we made it is 1 hour 45 minutes 20 seconds. "I'm going to have a couple of glasses of wine after this to celebrate," said Kerry, and the little lass from Scunthorpe headed off to be with her family.

Eventually, I found my way back to the car and got it started. But while we were waiting in a queue in the muddy grass field, straw caught on the axle and smoke was beginning to pour from the underside of my vehicle. It wasn't quite alight, but it was getting there, so having turned off the ignition I managed to scramble under the car, pull some of the straw clear, and gingerly move the car off the straw and away. What a day!

41. June 27th: Army Orienteering Association race @ Longmoor Camp, Hampshire.

HERE was a first for me. The first time I had ever competed in a race to be greeted by heavily armed soldiers at the gate, and then during the run itself to be accompanied by the sound of gunfire.

No, it wasn't the Baghdad Half Marathon but the Longmoor Training Camp just north of Petersfield in Hampshire. The area around Bordon and Longmoor has been used as an Army training camp since the 19th century when the land was bought by the War Department in the mid 1880s. The Longmoor and Bordon areas are the historic home of railway soldiers. The original railway line was built to move a complete camp from Longmoor to Bordon in the early 1900s. From this relatively minor start, the British Army's railway transport system was built and played a hugely important role during the Second World War.

Within the Longmoor Training Area, there is a Second World War memorial near the site where the pilot, Richard Pryce-Hughes, was killed on April 15th, 1942; his damaged bomber crashed when he guided it away from the local residential area. The army centre was disbanded in 1969 and today the camp is primarily used by cadets.

It was those heavily-armed cadets who were strutting around in their khaki uniforms brandishing rifles when I turned up with a friend, Julian Lyne to compete in an Army orienteering event. Julian, who belongs to

Southampton Orienteering Club, is an old hand at the sport who has been on the run with a map since 1993.

"I had been acting as transport manager for my son Alex for a couple of years when I decided to give the sport a go, rather than just sit in the car park with the Sunday papers," explained Julian. "I did easy courses for a few months to get some confidence before tackling the grown up stuff. The early objective was to get home in time for tea!

"It took a long time to get any real consistency in my performance, several years, and even now I still make mistakes due to lack of concentration. The main difference now is that these errors cost me a lot less time than they used to, 20 minutes lost on a single leg was not that much of a rarity in the nineties, but now I get really cheesed off if a mistake costs me more than two or three minutes."

Julian, who was 63 that summer, reckoned he had knocked off two stone in weight through the sport. "I am still losing weight now, but very slowly," he added. The downside is the rate of injuries, and Julian's tale of woe from orienteering reads like an episode of TV's "Casualty".

"I managed to stay pretty well clear of injury until late 2003, when I sustained a major ankle injury; nerve, tendon, cartilage, and minor bone damage without actually breaking or dislocating anything properly. I still get some discomfort if I run over 6km. I usually overdosing on painkillers before a major race, and then the reaction is delayed until about the Tuesday!"

He had an appendicitis in March 2006, and a knee injury just a few months before we met. "One broken bone per year amongst the regular orienteers in the club seems to be about the norm," he added.

I wanted to include orienteering within the project to demonstrate the range of different running events. The problem is, I can't read a map! Give me a compass, and I'm all over the place. I asked whether I could bring a SatNav with me, but was told that was no use at all. So we were at Longmoor for one of a regular summer series of races, and I was going to shadow Julian on one of the novice courses.

It was a time trial, and when we turned up there were competitors milling about deciding which of the five different events they would compete in.

The races are graded according to difficulty. The harder the course, the less detail you get on the map which is given to you. On our menu of options was a 4km brown/blue course, a 4.1km event known as the Corridor, a No Paths race over 5km and a 1km event called the Line. The aim was to navigate your way to one of the many control points hidden along the course, which were marked by an orange and white control kite. Each runner carries an electronic key with them, which is laid flat at each control point to record their time.

For the novice course, which was spread over 3.8km and described as medium/difficult, we had 10 control points to work our way around. I carried a map with me, a map with different coloured shadings and marks, and the 10 control points marked. Julian carried the e-card, known in the sport as 'a brick' which he inserted at each of the controls. It's a far cry from the pre-electronic days of orienteering, when runners would carry pieces of 6x3 inch cards marked with numbered square boxes which were known as control cards. At each control site there was a pin punch like a big pair of tweezers to register you had found the mark.

The problem was to find them. This was the first, and probably only time in my 80 race challenge when I competed in an event and I wasn't in control. I was entirely in Julian's hands. He had the map and compass, he knew what he was doing. I tried to follow the course from the map, holding the map in the direction we were heading and trying to pick out features.

More than once, I was jogging along trying to fix a point on the map and Julian was off, cutting across a ditch and over the heather. We had a dodgy start trying to find the first control point, but thereafter we seemed to ease our way around, criss-crossing other competitors. There was no point following them because they could be tracing another course.

I was surprised at how quickly Julian moved between the control points. A good 20 years older than me, he was still swift of foot, and managed to cut a fast swathe through the clinging heather, and through heavily forested areas. One of Julian's mottos is that the best way of orienteering quickly is to know when to go slowly. Another is never get yourself lost in the circle of uncertainty. I'd like to remember that mantra, but I'm not so sure!

I was a passenger on this run, trying to keep up with my partner over the hilly and barren terrain - jumping over tank tracks, detouring round barbed wire, looking up at the circling helicopters and listening to the cacophony of gunfire in the distance. Eventually, we found the tenth checkpoint, Julian inserted the electronic key, and we then moved swiftly to the finish. It took us 35 minutes 2 seconds for the distance. We probably covered about 4.5km.

It was a little anti-climactic since once we had finished, we then trotted off to the car to change and wait for one of Julian's friends, Robin, to finish. In the end we were placed ninth from a field of 45, some seven minutes behind the winner, which was fairly good.

"Orienteering is definitely addictive," added Julian. "I get withdrawal symptoms if I don't get to events on a regular basis. I think it's the lure of completing that elusive perfect run. I would guess that I've done about 500 events over the years, and I can recall only two that came anywhere near close.

"When people ask me why I run, I tell them, there's not really a reason, it's just the adrenalin when you start, and the feeling when you cross that finish line, and know that you are a winner no matter what place you got."

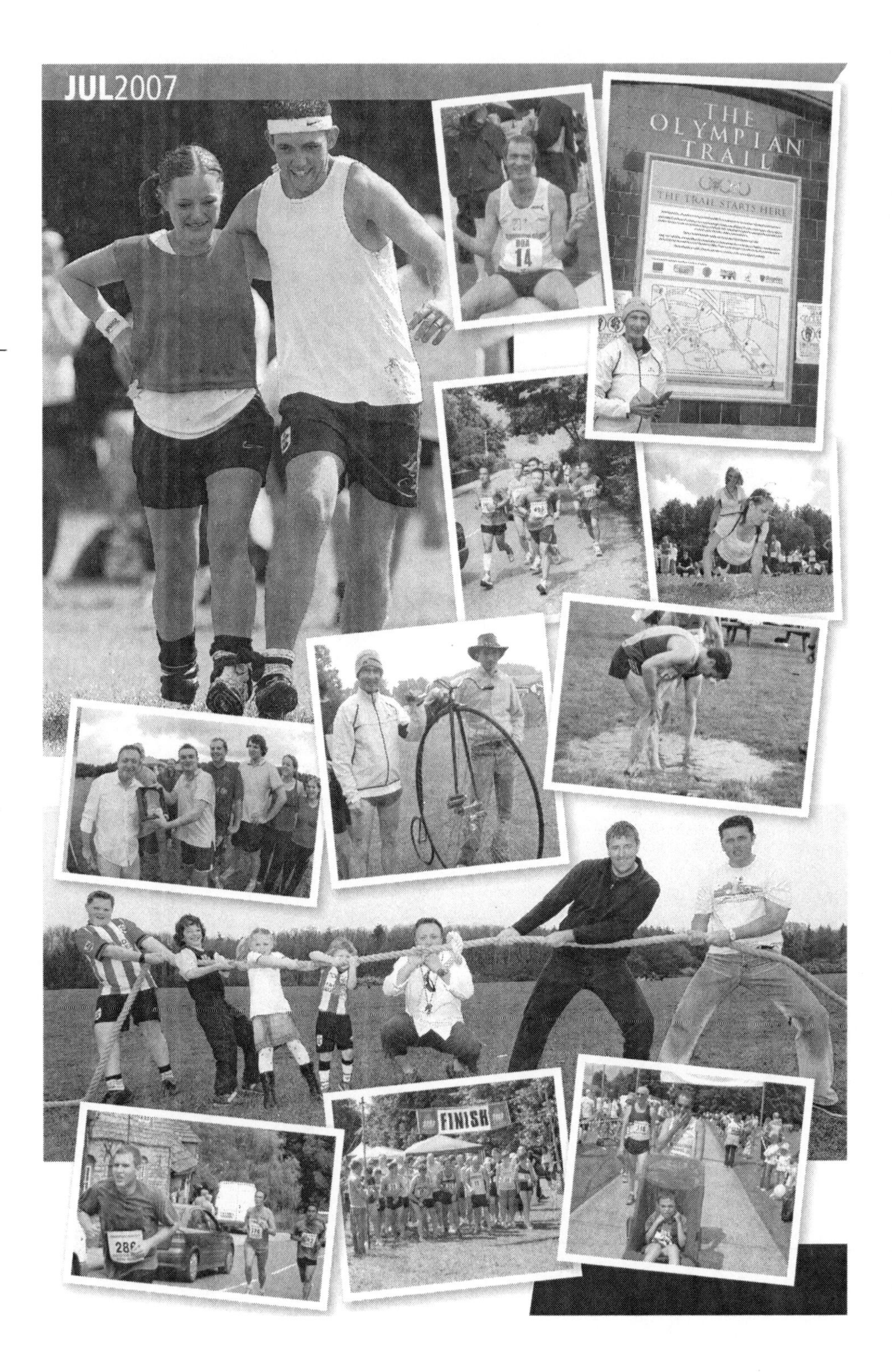
JUL2007
THE OLYMPIAN TRAIL
THE TRAIL STARTS HERE
FINISH

JULY

42. Prestwood 10k @ Leicestershire

THE worst thing which can ever happen to a runner apart from the injury, falling down a pothole in the middle of the road or being struck by a light plane, is when the call of nature strikes.

Inevitably before a race your body is hydrated with more water than would fill the Dead Sea. Just look at the long queues outside the portable toilets minutes before the start to see the huge number of runners who need to go for a quick constitutional.

Within the first mile of the London Marathon there is a bank of loos where it is incredible to see the number of folk who suddenly veer off course so early in the race and go straight for a leak.

Before each race, I stick to the same routine; Weetabix or sweet porridge for breakfast with a huge mug of sweet tea. Then, as I change an hour before the run, I grab a high-energy chocolate bar, drink a bottle of Lucozade and go through a few stretches. I can't abide with all those intensive pre-race workouts. Sometimes you see runners going out for a couple of kilometres' warm-up an hour before the start. Not for me, because if I did I would be totally pooped before the race. A few years ago I picked up a great tip to prevent a mid-race loo crisis which was to take Immodium an hour before a race. It is brilliant. Okay, it is a tablet used for diahorrea, but next to plugging a cork up your backside, it doesn't half stop the need for number twos.

So with the trip to Leicestershire for race 42, it was the same pre-race preparation as before for the 10km around a disused airfield. After the back to back sequence of June half marathons, which take a hell of a lot out of you physically, it was a relief to step into a race which was a lot less gruelling or pressurised.

The Prestwold Hall 10km was a new event organised by Barrow Runners in Leicestershire. For years they had hosted a 10-mile race, but after runners complained the race was too hot and hilly, and whinged about the ever-increasing traffic problems, that forced a rethink. What a shame, because at the risk of trying to compromise, Barrow Runners have probably come up with one of the most boring courses possible.

The 10km race is staged at Prestwold, a disused airfield and now a racetrack, situated just outside of Loughborough. It used to be known as Wymeswold Airfield, and home to the RAF from 1942 to 1978. During the Second World War, thousands of aircrews trained at Wymeswold which was home to a wing of Wellingtons, Lancasters, Stirlings and Halifaxes.

With most of the races taking place on a Sunday for this round Britain tour, I've chosen either to drive to the event on the morning of the race while the milkman is doing his rounds, which is tough – or for the very long trips to stay overnight in an hotel or bed & breakfast which have varied in quality.

On this first weekend in July, I managed to bag an invitation to stay with some friends Doug and Sally who own a pretty cottage in the back of beyond in the Leicestershire countryside. Liz and my youngest son Ross came with me. I wanted to give Ross only his second run out in the specially-adapted sports stroller which had been given a successful debut in Battersea Park the previous month.

This was the one advantage of racing around such a boring course on a disused airfield; it was relatively flat and easy to push my six-stone son around without too much discomfort. The race organisers had given me race number one, but we taxied to the back of the field as we prepared for the start on the main runway.

There had been flooding from the banks of the nearby River Soar and heavy overnight rain led to a feeling that we would get soaked. But fortunately the rain clouds held off just until the end of the race.

The race route was made up of a figure of eight around the old airfield. I stayed with Liz pushing Ross along and enjoying the slower pace. However Liz found the run a struggle; it was just one of those days for her.

For me it was good to step off the gas, to give Ross a good run out and to chat with other runners as we ambled along. It did get a little tougher towards the end pushing Ross. Imagine running with your hands held out in front of you for an hour and pushing at the same time. It is not easy. You don't realise how much you tend to rely on your arms for forward momentum. Ultimately, all the power and the pushing were coming from my legs.

Ross was dressed with a poncho covering him to catch the showers. He sat there, often with his hands pushed to his ears in the classic autism pose. His face was blank – it didn't tell anyone whether he was enjoying himself, or suffering. Selfishly, I wanted Ross to be part of this running voyage of discovery. He wouldn't be able to take part in a lot of races, but since the challenge's aim was to spread the word about autism here was the very real face of that disability. The face of an angel who was locked in his cotton wool world.

We managed to finish the 10km in 58 minutes 15 seconds, well outside Liz's personal best, but another race ticked off my list. Good race mementos from the organisers of a paperweight and a pack of cards!

Interestingly enough, to run in Leicestershire I had been forced to turn down an interesting invitation to race in Wales. The Tything Barn 5km was the last race of what organisers described as "a unique sporting event". This was a running race for naturists!

Earlier in the year, I had been contacted by the same organisers to run in another naturist running race in Kent called Naked Ambition. "The spectacular 25-acre site at Tything Barn in Pembrokeshire is an ideal venue for what is probably the finest clothing-optional running event in the UK," said the race literature for the Welsh run. "Although the pathways are in good order, the surface is uneven in places and runners should take care. Trail shoes are strongly recommended."

I was seriously keen to take part at Tything Barn and would have definitely run in the pink and crinkly – for scientific reasons, of course – had I not been committed to the Prestwood 10km. Ian Murray, my editor in Southampton, wanted me to take video coverage of the race, but I thought a headcam was a saucy step too far. I wonder where they pin the race numbers and don't even talk about chafing?!

43. Tickhill Gala Run @ Doncaster, South Yorkshire.

THE drama happened in a matter of seconds. It was early morning on a crisp, clear day driving along the M27 between Portsmouth and Southampton. In front, driving in the middle lane, was a pick-up truck with a canoe strapped to the back, its nose perched on the roof of the cab. I was following behind in my car with my three sons sat in the back on our way to Yorkshire – Ross was enjoying his Thomas the Tank engine DVD, Micah and Leo were reading as we hurtled down the motorway at 70mph.

Suddenly, the truck in front gently swerved from one side to the next, almost playfully. Seconds later, the swerve became jerkier and then the driver lost control.

The van flipped towards the hard shoulder, somersaulting three times over the Tarmac and into some vegetation before coming to rest high on a tree-covered bank. I quickly pulled over to the hard shoulder, grabbed my mobile phone and ran out of the car to help. What a muppet. I had left my three boys in the car, unprotected. Quickly, I re-traced my steps, got the boys out of the car, sat them on the bank and told them to wait.

I called the emergency services running the 100 metres to the smouldering wreckage with steam rising out of the bonnet. Surely no-one could have survived such a high-speed spill. Yet remarkably when I got to the truck it had landed on its wheels, the front windscreen was shattered and there was the driver, her face bloodied but conscious. Incredibly, she was fumbling for her phone to make a call. I tried to release the passenger side door – she was trapped on the other side – but the door was buckled and wouldn't budge.

I was soon joined by two guys who were landscape gardeners. They brought some shovels with them, and we managed to smash open the window. "I'm fine, I'm fine," called out the driver, clearly in shock and bleeding. I had brought water with me, tissues and wet wipes which I handed to her. The emergency services took an age to arrive. A couple of very bolshy police officers who had not been to diplomatic school turned up, the ambulance was another five minutes in arriving. They managed to get the lady safely out of the vehicle and whisked her off to hospital. She'd had an amazing escape with just cuts to her face, a wrecked truck, and a canoeing holiday ruined.

My boys were fine when I rejoined them and we headed on our way north for two races in two days at country shows; one in South Yorkshire and the other in Lincolnshire.

At Tickhill on Saturday afternoon for the Tickhill Gala Run, there were just 44 runners for the 3.5-mile canter along craggy lanes and roads around the Yorkshire town which lies near Doncaster. Our three o'clock race was squeezed between the fancy dress judging and a shoot-out in the main ring by the Doncaster Gunslingers – a motley bunch of golden oldies who enjoy dressing up as cowboys.

But that's what made this running adventure so interesting, so contrasting. A few months ago I was running with 35,000 other folk through the streets of London, and now in early July I was going elbow to elbow with just 44 runners beside flood-damaged fields in this tiny South Yorkshire town.

Historically, Tickhill's presence goes back as far as 1066 when William the First gave lands to Roger de Busli, who administered them as the Honour of Tickhill. Today, it is a lively village boasting an 11th century castle, a duck pond, a fine church dating from the 15th century, and a number of public houses.

In the summer, the Scouts and Guides Association organise the Tickhill Gala when the parade though the village includes floats and the Gala Queen. There was still strong evidence of the floods which had caused havoc and death in this part of northern England when a month's rain had fallen in one day. Though the flood waters had subsided, sandbags still littered parts of the streets and tide marks could be seen on the sides of homes which had been flooded a week earlier.

At least the weather was hot, offering these folk some respite. For me, the warm temperatures on a humid afternoon drained the legs and it was an effort to get a decent pace. I finished 14th in a time of 25 minutes 14 seconds, which was just over seven-minute-mile pace. Micah, Leo and Ross were waiting at the finish, having used the time to demolish the tenner I'd given them for the various rides and stalls while I was running.

That afternoon, we drove towards Scunthorpe – the birthplace of Tony Jacklin, Donald Pleasance and Joan Plowright, and the home of Scunthorpe United – one of only three England professional football clubs with a rude word in their names. The Corus steel works on the edge of town are an eye sore. It's ironic that Scunthorpe used to be known as 'The Industrial Garden Town' on the grounds that it had a bigger area of parks, gardens, woodland per capita than any other town in England. It's not where I would choose to live, but served to provide a place to stay before the following day's fun.

44. Spilsby Show 6 @ Spilsby, Lincolnshire.

THE market town of Spilsby lies between the Lincolnshire Wolds and the Fens, not far from Boston. For more than 700 years it has been a market place for farmers and growers selling a variety of fresh local vegetables, livestock, meat and bread.

In the town you will find the Franklin House Bakery with a plaque to denote the birth place of the Lincolnshire explorer Sir John Franklin; a statue of the man dominates the market place. Sir John is often referred to as the man who ate his boots. For in 1819, while commanding his first expedition to the Arctic, he and his companions suffered incredible hardship and survived by eating lichen and leather from their boots.

The Spilsby Show is a grander affair than the Tickhill Gala and can trace its roots back to 1880. The Spilsby Gala was originally held in July when among the attractions was maypole dancing – strange! It has had several fits and starts in its history, but the show was revived in 1974 and today is a bustling and busy show with a main parade ring featuring displays of shire horses, a dog show, even a parade of British Legion veterans. It was a very busy show, with scores of fairground attractions and sideshows.

Stuart Craggs, who organised the race, was its first winner back in 1998 when it was held as a six-mile fun run. "We had a whopping entry of about 12 for that first race," recalled Stuart. "It was certainly fun - or funny - as only the first three ran the correct course while the rest of the field took a half mile shortcut - unintentionally I'm sure.

"The show was cancelled in 2001 due to the foot and mouth outbreak, but since then race numbers have gradually increased every year. . "At this rate we should reach 500 entries sometime around the middle of the century," added Stuart.

For the Spilsby race I decided to run with Ross in his sports stroller. Beforehand I had seen the course consisted of roads and bridleways so thought it would be okay to get Ross round. What I hadn't accounted for was just how tough it was going to be. The bridleways were bumpy and lumpy which must have given Ross a horrendous ride. It was tricky to push or to get any sort of momentum going. Along a rutted bridleway, I was forced to swerve between the pot holes trying to find good ground.

Ross was a happy bunny in the sunshine. He was chortling away cheered on by passing runners. After racing in the countryside, there was a nice downhill stretch back into Spilsby for the finish in the showground.

We finished towards the back of the field. I came 74th out of 116 runners with a time of 48min 59sec which was a pretty poor time as I had covered the first open mile-long stretch in a stonking seven minutes, but after that it was a slog.

The one consolation of being a tail-ender was that I was able to test out my totally unscientific theory that the prettier the female, the slower the runner. Of course, this is a purely subjective theory which has no mathematical correlation, but which through exhaustive research built up over a number of years, consistently runs true to form and which was proved so at Spilsby.

Towards the back of a race field, you will find some absolute corkers. Carefree spirits with an easy running style, looking pretty cool in their designer gear. They may be slow, but they are pleasing to the eye, some running with Ipods, others running with barely a bead of sweat on their forehead. Of course there are a few exceptions to the rule who ought to be wearing signs on their backsides saying "slow moving heavy load, please pass".

That's not to suggest that the fleet-footed females at the front of a race are lacking in the beauty department, it's simply that in my exhaustive research you will find the majority of the cream of the crop nestled neatly towards the rear. Oooh err!

All this science offers a crumb of comfort for me as I get slower, because at least I will have something to look forward in the autumn of my running career lumbering along at the back of a race field!

Anyway, as for Spilsby, once I had finished ogling the delightful ladies while pushing Ross in his stroller, I got back to find Micah and Leo had cleaned me out for yet another tenner on the fairground attractions.

This weekend had provided a very different slice of running life to the one I had been used to. The atmosphere at both Spilsby and Tickhill was far less intense and quite laid back – and for my boys it gave them a chance to see at close hand what the running challenge was all about.

45. Wenlock Olympian Games @ Shropshire.

MENTION the name of Much Wenlock and it's hard to imagine how this small Shropshire town could have a major impact on the sporting world - but it has. In fact, many would claim that it's thanks to Much Wenlock, a stone's throw from Shrewsbury, that the modern Olympic Games came into being.

William Penny Brooks who came from the town was an ardent advocate of physical education in schools. In 1850 he formed the Olympian class to "promote the moral, physical and intellectual improvement" of the good folk of Wenlock. He did this by starting up a sports day with a mixture of athletics and old country sports, such as cricket, football and quoits.

Dr Brookes' big dream was to revive the ancient Olympic Games, and in 1889 Baron de Coubertin visited the Wenlock Olympian Games. During his visit to Much Wenlock, Brookes shared his ideas for an international Olympic Games with the young French aristocrat. This inspired Coubertin to set up a conference at the Sorbonne where he organised a revival of the ancient Olympic Games. Sadly, Brookes died in 1895, just four months before the revived modern Olympic Games were first held in 1896 in Athens.

But his name lives on and the Wenlock Olympian Society has held a sporting festival in the village ever since. This year saw the staging of the 121st annual Wenlock Olympian Games with bowls, tennis, badminton, triathlon, fencing, archery, clay pigeon shooting, five-a-side football, volleyball, cricket, cycling, golf and....wait for it...a seven-mile road race.

When I arrived in the midlands, the rain was sheeting it down. The sodden summer continued unabated. The poor athletics competitors on the cinder track were drenched, and meanwhile officials had all sorts of problems getting cars parked on the school playing fields.

As for the road race, the runners took cover from the incessant downpour in a tea hut, under trees or in their cars until the sounding of a shrill whistle five minutes from the start. We lined up with the rain soaking through our clothes. I had been off work for most of the previous week with 'flu. For the first 400 metres I felt great, for the remaining 6.8 miles I felt dreadful! Runners cruised past me until I settled in midfield playing hare and tortoise with one runner who was rubbish going up hills but then tore past me going downhill.

A succession of hills came and passed a route which circled the Shropshire town before finally dropping downhill and running through the picturesque surroundings with its Tudor homes and narrow streets. For me, this race was about surviving. Ordinarily I would have skipped running at Much Wenlock because I was not well, but this was one race which is so steeped in history that it had to be among the select band of 80 races.

The last mile was a switchback through some woods and back onto the school playing fields to the finish. I managed to sprint ahead of the hare having eked out a lead with the final uphill stretch. Wet and weary, I trooped back to the car, glad I had packed a towel in my sports bag.

46. Mug's Game 5 @ Itchen Valley Country Park, Eastleigh, Hampshire.

THE date of Saturday, July 21st had been in the diary since late last summer since I always had in mind that I would organise one of the 80 races planned for the 2007 challenge and so the Mug's Game 5 was born.

For the past nine months I had been piecing together this 4.5-mile race around Itchen Valley Country Park near Eastleigh. The park nestles within earshot of Southampton Airport but provides a secluded and safe setting for a race. Unlike my involvement with the Stubbington 10km race earlier this year, there was no need for policing or road closures. This was a mixture of parkland and woodland, with a short stretch of Tarmac thrown in.

The race organisation was a huge undertaking, stitched together with all the running round the country, and the necessary financial diversion of holding down paid employment! The task was not helped by the stupid idea of ambitiously organising an old-style school sports day and traditional summer fete to run alongside the race. Why set yourself an easy task when you can make it harder?

Both events were in aid of the Hampshire Autistic Society which was fundamentally what this year was all about. Yes, it was about getting some decent exercise, clocking up quite a few miles in the car while seeing the four corners of the British Isles, but the bottom line was about raising money and awareness for the society. As the year progressed, so the racing and ultimately writing this book became secondary in importance. The running was a means to an end, a thread to hold the whole project together; the book was a nice way of wrapping up the package. But for me the work I was doing with the society, creating awareness about autism and its impact, was of the utmost importance.

Suddenly the need to generate media awareness about the challenge in newspapers, magazines, on radio and even grabbing the occasional couple of minutes on local television became a priority. I was hitting the phone and e-mailing media contacts all over the country where I would be running in the hope of grabbing a few column inches in the newspaper, or a few seconds on the radio. And it worked; BBC, independent local radio, regional newspapers, weekly papers. I had a few local champions too. Jon Cuthill on BBC Radio Solent, and Steve Power, the breakfast show presenter on Wave

105 on the south coast were just brilliant by frequently giving me airtime on their programmes.

As a Brucie bonus shortly before the sports day, I managed to get a three minute spot on the peak-time Meridian Tonight programme. Sarah Gomme, who I used to work with at the Southern Daily Echo, interviewed me at one of the Hampshire Autistic Society schools and then her cameraman took some general shots of me running up and down Southampton Common. Three minutes, 180 seconds, but at 6.20pm on a Thursday evening just as everyone was sitting down having their tea, it was simply perfect. Commercially, that would have cost hundreds of thousands of pounds to buy that air time and to plant those subliminal messages into viewers' minds about autism.

Together, with Sally Hillyear fundraising manager with the Hampshire Autistic Society we began giving talks to Rotary clubs, schools, business clubs, in fact anyone who wanted to hear a half-hour chat about the unlikely twin combination of autism and running. Chalk and cheese as subjects, but the combination seemed to strike a chord.

Sally and I have known each other for several years becoming the best of friends. We both share an interest in autism, and for me Sally provided much of the momentum behind the running challenge. A year earlier, we had shared a lunchtime picnic when I revealed my plans to run around the British Isles in 80 races in tandem with a major fund-raising project for the Hampshire Autistic Society.

Working with Sally at the Hampshire Autistic Society was Gemma Harvey, a gem of a lady who I first met when I was judging a beauty contest where she was one of the entries. She came third at that competition, but at the second time of bidding with Sally assisting me with the judging, Gemma was crowned Miss Winchester. A year or so later, Gemma, a 5ft 11in leggy blonde, joined the society as one of Sally's fund-raising team. The third member was Kerry James, a lady who I first met at a casino evening she was organising and where I had to carry Sally to the car after she became a little tipsy. She must have been impressed by Sally's alcohol intake because she too soon joined the team of three wise ladies. And what a team they are.

They were central to the organisation of the big day at Itchen Valley. The girls managed to persuade FoneTrader Business to sponsor the event. I had twisted the arms of Asics, and my friend Pete Staunton from the JustRun sports shop in Eastleigh to help me with much of the equipment for the race. I then gathered a team of friends to help me – Liz, along with Malcolm Price and Eryl Penney from Southampton Running Club, plus Stubbington Green Runner friends Nick and Helen Kimber, Paul and Marj Hammond. We planned together, agonised together, and worked together towards this day.

Despite the heavy media promotion, the response to both the sports day and the running race was painfully slow. It was not helped by the awful weather of the previous six weeks; rain, rain and still more numbingly, predictable rain. As a result, few people were prepared to commit to the fund-raiser. When I planned the date last summer, I felt the odds would be on my side for the weather; how wrong could I be? I should have never consulted the BBC weatherman Ian McCaskill about the prospects of a sun-drenched summer!

Come Saturday, by the time I opened my curtains at 6am the omens looked good; blue skies and bright sunshine. I drove to Itchen Valley with my dad for a walk around the running course, trimming back a few branches with a pair of secateurs. Though the woodland section was a little boggy, the ground underfoot was not too bad. The rest of the day went by in a blur, and with it the weather deteriorated. As the sports day teams pulled up in an assortment of vehicles the showers set in. It was miserable, and hard to keep a smile on your face.

For the old style sports day, I had press-ganged Brian Richardson, a Royal Navy physical training instructor based at HMS Temeraire in Portsmouth to organise the event.

Brian's claim to fame was that he once appeared as a contestant in the hit ITV show Gladiators. Now being revived in 2008 by Sky, this was a time when contenders took on the likes of Jet, Scorpio and Wolf.

Brian, who retired from the Navy at the end of 2007, told me how simply getting onto the televised show was as tough as the arena events.

London Weekend Television would receive around 22,000 applications for each series, and 16,000 hopefuls were invited to try out with just 36 contenders making it on prime-time Saturday evening television. The hopefuls had to run 800 metres on a treadmill in under 2 minutes 30 seconds for a man, and under three minutes for a woman. They had a two minute break before moving onto the straight arm pull-ups. Each contender had to hang by their arms from a horizontal bar with an underhand grip and pull their body up so that their chin was above the bar. The men had to do 10 chin-ups, the women had to complete five.

A minute later, the test was to traverse a 15 foot monkey ladder and then climb a 20 foot rope before carefully lowering themselves. Women had to do this exercise once within a minute. Men had to climb the rope twice, again within 60 seconds. No rest was allowed between the ladder and the rope. And that wasn't it. If the would-be contender had made it to this point, it was now time for a pugil stick fight to test their aggression. For 30 seconds one contender would attack, while the other defended. The positions were then reversed with a 30 second rest between bouts.

Brian was not a man you wanted to fall out with. Actually, he was a thoroughly nice guy who on the day brought along with him a couple of trainee Navy PTIs to put the ten teams through their paces in games such as three-legged races, a sack race, egg and spoon and even a ski race. My mate Steve Power did his best to whip up enthusiasm on the microphone, but the afternoon's games were dogged by showers. It was not pleasant. The stalls were doing hardly any trade, but fair play to the sports day competitors who threw themselves about in the rain.

Inwardly, I felt so dejected. Months of planning had gone into a day which had turned on the unseasonable weather. It was a damp squib. I managed to see a little bit of the sports day while working with the rest of the team to get the course set for the running race. Eastleigh Air Cadets were safely ushering in a stream of cars, St John Ambulance were on standby, and the wonderful park rangers led by Rachel Odell were pitching in.

Come race time, a good-sized crowd of a hundred or so runners had turned up, the showers had disappeared, and the sun was shining. One kilometre and two kilometre children's races were held beforehand which passed off peacefully but for one parent who was unhappy her child hadn't received the correct prize. And then at 6pm, 108 runners took part in the first-ever Mug's Game 5. I was so delighted when Malcolm Price sounded the starting horn and the race was under way.

The multi-lap race was based on grassland and woodland providing a tricky test. It was won by the talented Chichester runner, James Baker, with Karen Rushton from Southampton Running Club claiming the ladies' race. There were a few pre-race hiccups, but everything seemed to go off well. Prizes were handed out efficiently, no-one got lost or was injured on the route, everyone seemed happy with the post-race drinks and fruit, and the atmosphere was a friendly one. Come 7pm and the finish of the race, I was feeling exhausted. I was acting as a gopher between the finish funnel and the results recorder, Richard Dean, who did an outstanding job.

As competitors and their families started to head home, so the heavens opened; and this as we began the process of packing away. Thankfully, many of the volunteers had stayed behind to assist, and despite a brief respite in the tent to hide from the showers, we were gone by 8pm. I still had a van to drop off, tables to clean to be left at the local church, and it wasn't until almost 10pm when I could shut the door behind me at home and collapse beside a plate of chilli.

It was a long day, but a very worthwhile one at that. The race alone raised almost £1,200. I'd over-ordered on the mugs big-time with several hundred sat in the back of my car. By the time expenses had taken care of, the sports day raised £2,500 profit and substantial awareness for autism.

I was due to run in Kent the following morning at the Dartford Half Marathon, which incidentally was won in its inaugural year by the former Olympic champion Steve Ovett, when the entry free was a measly 30 pence. However, to get to one of Kent's longest-running races would have required a 5.30am wake-up call to get there for a 9am start. So I slept through the obscenely early alarm call and instead spent the day at home.

47. Swanage Half Marathon @ Swanage, Dorset.

YOU don't meddle with the Gurkhas, not unless you want to get hurt. The Nepalese soldiers have been serving the British crown since 1815 and have fought with distinction in conflicts across the world.

These guys are hard. Each year, from a training camp in Pokhara in the foothills of the Himalayas and the Annapurna mountain range, 230 young men are recruited for the British Army after rigorous selection.

Just as a guide, in regional selection the young recruits have to run 800 metres in under two minutes and 40 seconds, perform 14 under-arm heaves hanging from a bar, and perform 70 sit-ups in just two minutes. Does this sound like Gladiators again?!

If they get through that physical test, the candidates then move on to central selection where they have to run 1.5 miles in under nine minutes 40 seconds, and complete a 5 kilometre route march with a 450 metre ascent while carrying a 25kg load in 48 minutes.

These guys are physically and mentally fit. "They're like machines. Give them a task and they will do it. They don't say much, but they are very single-minded and bloody hard." Those were the wise words of Scouser who was running beside me at the Swanage Half Marathon. He was a private with the Royal Signals based at the same Dorset camp as the Gurkhas.

We were four miles into the race which proved to be a gruelling test through the beautiful, undulating Dorset countryside. It traced a route through the Purbecks on the north side of Nine Barrow Down. The road to Corfe Castle is tough to run; a never-ending sequence of crunching climbs enveloped by a baking sun. For the six Gurkhas from the Queen's Gurkha Signals, dressed in khaki tops and shorts, this was a breeze.

Just as I was chatting to the Scouser, the Gurkhas suddenly pushed on and I stupidly tried to go with them. For the next half hour, these tiny fellas ate up the miles. I towered over them and occasionally they would look behind to see where I was. I tried a few bits of conversation, but there were no replies. Nothing was said, they clinically pushed on. All I could do was to stick close on their heels and right on their pace.

At Corfe Castle, where the ruins were clad in scaffolding and sheeting, the two front-running Gurkhas decided to make a break from their colleagues. They surged up the hill on a rising bend and I did something stupid – I went with them. Now I'm not a bad hill climber and more than held my own as we left behind the four other Gurkhas, but by the top of the rise I was beat. The two Nepalese privates kicked on at the top of the climb where I was left isolated.

The arduous efforts of the past four miles had left me drained. Though the second half of the race was less torrid with the route running back through the valley to Swanage, I was grimly hanging on. At every water stop I took on as much liquid as possible but my legs had no power in them whatsoever. Someone had switched off the batteries. Thank heavens for the downhill run into the seaside town which was buzzing because this was carnival weekend.

I managed to keep ahead of the other Gurkhas, though I sensed they would pass at any time. At the finish I finally caught up with the two leading soldiers sitting on a wall by the beach. They looked so relaxed and had hardly broken sweat. "That was fun," said Ajib, just 20-years-old, relaxing with his mate Sanjaykumar, who had finished five minutes ahead of me.

"What about the hills?" I asked. "We have bigger hills back home!" they replied. I thought the guys were taking the mick, but then I wasn't going to argue with a Gurkha!

As for the race, the Swanage Half Marathon proved to be a tough, but enjoyable one. It is reckoned to be one of the oldest country road races in the UK.

"We do not know the exact date of when the race was started but we do know of local men who won it in the early 1900s," explained Linda Welch, the Swanage Regatta & Carnival Secretary.

"My own opinion is that this race was started for the local stone workers, in those days, the biggest employment was in the stone quarries and I could well imagine that this was a competition between the local stonemasons.

"The beautiful silver cup we have was presented in 1927 by Russell Parsons Esq to the Swanage British Legion and inscribed as a Marathon Race Trophy. This suggests that in those days the race was held for ex-military men if the British Legion ran it.

"My recollections of the race going back to the late 50s and early 60s were always of just men entering. They had to run past the house I lived in and we would sit outside to watch, certainly in those days, no women entered."

In the early 1990s and until 2005 the race was known as the Swanage 12. But for the past two years, the organisers added the extra mile. "That extra mile which takes the course to Studland has added a sting in the tail," explained one wiry-looking runner, who has made the event an annual pilgrimage.

He wasn't wrong. After weeks and weeks of incessant rain, trust the weather to put his hat on big style. It was a boiler for a gruelling test through the beautiful, undulating Dorset countryside.

The race began in the seaside town on the first day of its carnival. The beach was busy, the fairground rides were attracting good business. I finished the half marathon in 1 hour 46 minutes, my slowest 13-miler of the year so far, so as I left the two Gurkhas to enjoy the seaside, I headed for the beach and a post-race dip in the still slightly cold waters of the English Channel.

"Running is a big question mark that's there each and every day. It asks you, 'Are you going to be a wimp or are you going to be strong today?'"

AUG2007

LANDS END 2007
NEW YORK 3147
JOHN O'GROATS 874
ISLES OF SCILLY 28
LONGSHIPS LIGHTHOUSE 1½
AROUND THE BRITISH ISLES IN 80 RACES

AUGUST

48. Harlow 10 @ Harlow, Essex.

IT was 83 degrees by the time I got back to the car at the end of the Harlow 10. It was hot, it was humid, it was the hottest day of the year.

I was shattered at the end of what I thought would be a gentle 10-miler around the Essex town. Thank heavens for the early 9.30am start because had the race time been much later in the day then conditions would have been even worse.

I had originally planned to run a 10km at Tenbury Wells in Worcestershire, an area which had been badly hit by the recent floods. I had e-mailed the race organisers to check whether the event was still on but had heard nothing. The thought of entering on the day and there not being a race was too risky. As it was the Tenbury 10km did go ahead in brilliant sunshine, even though parts of the course had been covered in six feet of water. Some runners had suggested on one of the web forums that they might need to bog snorkel to the finish since conditions were so bad.

After a pitiful run at Swanage the previous week, I reckoned what I needed was some distance in my legs. There was not much to choose from race-wise in the first week of August and so the Harlow 10 beckoned.

I had not been to Harlow for 25 years from the time when I spent a year there training as a journalist at the town's technical college. Back in 1981, it was the first time I had left the comforts of home to set out on the road of journalism. I found lodgings in a two-bedroom semi owned by a 70-year-old Coronation Street-loving grandmother by the name of Rachel Horton. She was lovely. What surprised me most about Rachel was her love for Dire Straits as she could regularly be found playing one of the group's albums on her old-style record player. Just picture the scene of her lip-synching to "Romeo and Juliet" and "Sultans of Swing". The reason for Rachel's love of Dire Straits was that one of her first lodgers from the journalism college had been Mark Knopfler, the group's lead singer. He studied at Harlow Technical College in 1967 and later went to work as a reporter for the Yorkshire Evening Post, before going on to greater things in the music world. Mark had stayed in touch with Rachel and every time Dire Straits released an album he would send a copy to her.

Ironically, a few years later I caught up with Mark when he was going through one of those expensive motor racing phases which all pop stars seem to need to experience as a rite of passage. We met at a cold and windswept Snetterton circuit in Norfolk. Mark was in a huffy mood not wanting to give any interviews, keeping away from the media throng. Eventually I sidled up to the great man since I was under strict orders from my editor to get an interview for my paper and opened with the line: "You and I have got something in common – do you remember Rachel Horton?" Suddenly his icy demeanor changed. We chatted about Rachel, compared notes on Harlow, and then went off for a quiet coffee where he gave me the interview.

I can't say that Harlow held too many cherished memories; cramming shorthand and law, going to the pub to play Phoenix and Space Invaders, lunchtime snooker at a club behind the town hall, and finding the first love of my life; a fellow journalist called Susan. The town used to smell of gin from the nearby Gilbey's distillery and its architecture was grim; typical of those 1950s London overspill towns. Harlow, in fact, celebrated its 60th birthday in 2007.

Twenty five years on and it was hard to compare Harlow from the 1980s to its 21st century version since the race didn't venture too near the town centre. Instead it started and finished at the recently-built Mark Hall Sports Centre taking a route which headed up to the town park and back. The lowlight of the race was a back-breaking and gruelling climb at mile eight. Ordinarily this would not have been a problem, but after a stamina-sapping run in the extreme heat it was tough and many runners were forced to walk up the sharp rise.

I hate running in the heat and had nothing to give. A few years ago, a friend had suggested we train together to compete in the epic Marathon des Sables – a six-day endurance race across the Sahara Desert for a total of 151 miles. I'd rather set fire to my hair and poke my eyes out with needles than enduring that Moroccan madness. Back in Harlow, I was counting the miles from the four mile mark. The race route wasn't that inspiring, though the marshals were there when it mattered with the drinks and sponge stations. My time of 1 hour 19 minutes was slow, very slow, but to be honest I was pleased to have got round.

That should have been my second run of the weekend since 24 hours earlier I had been driving up the M3 to compete in the Bushy Park time trial at Hampton Court in Middlesex. This is a popular 5 kilometre run held every Saturday morning and is extremely highly-rated by runners everywhere. I would run at Bushy Park later in the year, but on this August day I had just started out on my early morning journey to south-west London when I heard on the radio that there had been a double death in Winchester involving a woman and her young child. I quickly turned round and headed back to the office to work on the next edition of the newspaper.

A few days after the Harlow run and the day before my trip to South Wales, I had a tough gig to attend in aid of the running project. I had to audition before the Women's Institute, the same trusted organisation of fearsome ladies who once gave Tony Blair a torrid time at their national conference a few years back.

This was the Hampshire WI who, a few times each year, hold auditions for speakers wanting to talk to their members around the county. You could describe it as the WI does X-Factor. I even paid a fee for the privilege of attending the audition and then £10 for an entry in the WI handbook if successful. Fellow WI members were invited to attend the auditions, and for this outing 43 ladies had turned up to the headquarters in Winchester to hear four speakers talk on a variety of subjects from press photography and the world of gastronomic delights, to adventures in Borneo and my subject... autism and running.

I was there with Sally from the Hampshire Autistic Society. As we were greeted by a lovely lady called Cherry, offered tea and small talk, I was bricking it. So too was Sally who admitted later that if we could have made a dignified exit then she would have – and I would have joined her. We could hear the laughter from upstairs where the Fleet Street photographer was in full swing. We didn't have too many laughs in our half-hour ditty.

At the appointed hour, a petite, silver-haired lady called Fearne met us and led us into the room where the fearsome-looking 43 ladies greeted us. It was intimidating. We had five minutes to set up, so Sally and I busied ourselves putting up a display, plugging in a computer and a projector for a five-minute film which we wanted to show at the end.

I am never normally edgy with public speaking, but it was the sight of those ladies clutching their pads of paper and pens and the fact they were judging us which was unnerving. They were no Simon Cowell, but this was so bizarre. When the lady in front row started scribbling some notes within seconds of Sally talking I thought "uh oh, we're dead in the water!"

In truth the talk went well as the ladies warmed to us. We got a few laughs; we also got some tears at the end from the video which I had put together with a friend from the BBC telling the story of autism through the eyes of Ross. It was an exhausting half hour, I was sweating badly by the time we left the room to make way for the talk from the flame-haired speaker about life in Borneo.

How did we do? Well, amazingly we got accepted, and during 2008 Sally and I have been doing a few WI talks in Hampshire.

49. Mynyddislwyn Mile @ Newbridge, South Wales.

THE Mynyddislwyn Mile: when you've run out of vowels that's one heck of a Scrabble choice on a triple word score! It was also the shortest, sharpest and nastiest race I endured in the quest to run around the British Isles in 80 races.

The event, organised by Islwyn Runners, is known as "The Mad Mile" or "The Murderous Mile". It is reputed to be the toughest mile race in Britain with a course record of seven minutes 50 seconds, so I knew this was going to be hellish. Driving across the congested Severn Bridge into Wales, I wondered what on earth I was doing driving all the way from the south coast for a one-mile race on a Friday evening. But I am so glad I did it.

The village of Mynyddislwyn lies in Ebbw Valley in Gwent, not far from Pontypool, a town made legendary by the rugby club's fearsome front row forwards of the 1970s; Anthony Faulkner, Bobby Windsor and Graham Price. The hamlet is surrounded by farmland, forest, and hills. Driving up a narrow, steep lane off the main road and into Mynyddislwyn gives you an idea of what lies in store.

This is a very relaxed and informal race. I parked at the top of the hill, and found the race organisers sat on a bench at the entrance to the old St Tudor Church and right next to the Church Inn where they were dishing out numbers and handing out safety pins.

Years ago, they explained, there had been a popular race called the Murder Mile in nearby Newport. It was a similarly stern test; a belt and braces run up the steepest of hills.

The race started in the 1990s serving as a small informal event. There were just 10 runners for the inaugural mile. But numbers have picked up in recent years as word has spread about its notoriety.

"The race it is in its 10th year and started when we did a Murder Mile that Newport Harriers promoted," explained Michael Heare from Islwyn Running Club. "We thought that with all the hills we have around the valleys we could find a tougher one.

"We ran up the Murder Mile in the middle of a 10-mile training run and we always had a bit of a race to see who could reach the top first, so we had it measured and organised a race. For the first few years just club members and a few guests ran the race, but last year we had over 50 entries."

The Mynyddislwyn Mile packs a mean one in eight gradient up this country lane bordered by trees and fields. The road is rutted in places and littered with stones, not making it the easiest of runs. Except for one short plateau midway through the torture, and then a gentle run-in with a slight downhill at the finish, the race is a sheer climb.

To get to the start there was a gentle jog of two miles from the church to the bottom of the hill. Thank God this wasn't a downhill race. Jogging to the start you could sense the steep gradient as your legs ran away from you.

Limbering up at the start, you could see the tension in everyone's face knowing what lay ahead. It may only be one mile, but this was going to hurt. "You're all mad!" shouted the organiser from the safety of his car, where he leant out of the window to give the countdown to the start before shooting up the hill in his vehicle ahead of the pack. How I would have laughed had the car stalled and the handbrake not worked!

This was a brutal run up a narrow lane. It was 7pm, and humid too. I started gently up the climb, but within a minute the hill was hurting and my pace was slowing. This was brutal. I was sweating profusely and breathing hard. The lactic acid was kicking in big time. One writer once described this race as "like a gruelling mountain stage of the Tour de France, but without the hooting, the Devil with his pitchfork running beside you, the French Police outriders or the Coca-Cola sponsor cars."

I try to tackle hills like climbing a set of stairs, keeping a rhythmic pattern to my steps, leaning into the rise while trying to relax. I looked at my watch and we were two minutes in. My hamstrings were screaming, a few runners eased past, my pace was slowing almost to a walk.

I wanted to run the whole way, but just before the half mile mark I knew this was pointless. I could speed walk faster than I could run by pushing off my knees with my hands. I felt ashamed to walk, but I had nothing left in my legs.

After the short plateau, the climb got even steeper. The three-quarter of a mile mark, which was chalked into the road, loomed large. My back was aching, my knees were hurting, my body was asking how much longer? I looked up and could see the hill level out, so I pushed myself for one final, big effort. It was nothing more than a jog, and once onto this level stretch of road I was able to open out a bit more. It was heavenly to finally run on a flat piece of ground, and the slight downhill at the end was absolute bliss.

Because of roadworks at the bottom of the hill, the course for 2007 had been slightly altered, but the race was won by Afan Humphries from Cwmbran in 7 minutes 34 seconds with Angela Jones from Brecon the leading lady in 9 minutes 25 seconds.

I crossed the finish line in a time of 12min 15sec – my slowest mile ever, to be greeted by the sight of water, plus bottles of beer and cider were being gratefully received by the runners.

The Myyddislwyn Mile is there to be conquered. In a sadistic sort of way, it was fun!

From South Wales, I drove straight to Birmingham because I had a morning flight to catch from the airport to the Isle of Man. I got totally lost in Brum trying to find my hotel and got pulled over by a couple of very good-looking female traffic cops.

"You were driving quite erratically, sir, we thought you might have been drinking," said one, as I sat in the back of their car. Get the handcuffs out, I thought! "Sorry to disappoint you, but I don't drink," I replied, as the other gorgeous uniformed gal was radioing through to check out the car registration and whether I had tax and insurance. "The bad driving was just down to being lost," I added, and with that the two lovely ladies sent me on my way with directions to the hotel. I slept well that night gripped by an x-rated dream involving Juliet Bravo and that fit-looking bird off The Bill!

50. Isle of Man Half Marathon.

RUNNING is a confidence thing. A week earlier I had suffered in the heat over ten miles at a race in Harlow. Afterwards I'd felt drained and dejected by my pitiful performance. I didn't enjoy the run one bit.

Seven days later on the Isle of Man, I finished the half marathon with a big smile on my face. Fortieth place in a time of 1 hour 38 minutes was very satisfactory – so much so that I had run the first 10 miles on the Isle of Man five minutes faster than I had in Essex. Running, it seems, is all about confidence.

The Isle of Man is a beautiful part of the world. Just 33 miles long and 13 miles wide, it has a rugged coastline not too dissimilar to Cornwall. The hinterland has a series of spectacular hills with the highest, Snaefell, which means Snow Mountain, standing at 2,036 feet.

The beauty of the Isle of Man is its charm, although one senses the place exists in something of a time warp. I stayed in a hotel looking out on Ramsey Bay just outside of the island's second largest town. The hotel had seen better days, but in its heyday was clearly the place to be. The hotel had a bit of a Fawlty Towers feel to it. The décor in the tiny single room was very 1970s. The television was almost as old as a crystal set. You had to play around with the aerial to get any sort of picture.

Ramsey, though, is a lovely place with its distinctive harbour, Victorian pier and Mooragh Park. The town has played a major role throughout the centuries of Manx maritime history and was once a centre for shipbuilding. Now tourism dominates, especially around the time of the TT motorbike races.

At the time, the big story on the island centred around the foot and mouth outbreaks on the mainland. For the Isle of Man, which is so dependent on agriculture, the authorities had decided to batten down the hatches. The headline on the front of the Isle of Man Examiner blasted: "Fortress Island". The Royal Manx Agricultural Show was cancelled; public footpaths were closed, as were some glens.

As I stepped off the Flybe flight from Birmingham, we were quizzed by Ministry of Agricultural officials whether we had been in contact with livestock on the mainland and if we intended to travel to a farm. They asked if we had bought any meat sandwiches with us. Before the half marathon we were warned not to take a leak on farmland because of the very real fear of spreading foot and mouth. "Vigilance has kept us foot-and-mouth free for 100 years," said the Examiner, and the islanders weren't going to allow any peeing runners to ruin that unblemished record.

Mind you, we could only have a tinkle after drinking liquid supplied by the organisers. One of the more bizarre pre-race instructions dictated that during the race we could only take liquid from drinks stations provided by the organisers. "This is to ensure that all athletes compete on a fair basis. i.e: one runner may not have the advantage over another by having family/ friends supplying drinks on demand – a facility which is not available to all competitors," said the organisers. How stupid and ridiculous, but apparently these are UK Athletics' rules.

The race itself started and finished at Ballacloan Stadium, the home of Ramsey Football Club. Stadium is perhaps too grand a word for the place which consisted of one stand where the changing rooms were sited and a small track down one side, which acted as a finishing straight.

This was two races in one with the marathon runners completing two laps of the 13-mile loop to our one, and starting off half an hour earlier. Unlike Harlow where temperatures had soared into the 80s, it was cloudy and raining for the start of both events, though as the races progressed so the clouds lifted and the sun shone. But it was still comfortable running weather for a tough hilly opening four miles which didn't allow you to settle on the coastal road to Bride overlooking the cliffs and magnificent beaches.

However once you turned off that road, so the route became flatter. I ran virtually alone but was able to enjoy the huge green expanse of hillside, with wispy crowds covering the peaks.

The country lanes to Andreas at seven miles were quiet where I picked off the first of the marathon runners who'd been given a half hour head start. I didn't envy them one bit with the long road which lay ahead of them. Several were members of the 100 Marathon Club, an elite band who have endured more than a century of 26-milers. I've done three and that is my lot!

Among those who completed the marathon was blind runner Paul Watts from Chestnut in Hertfordshire, who is a member of Barnet & District AC. The 42-year-old was running with guides Steve Price and Colin Longworth from Liverpool AC, eventually completing the distance in just over five hours. Paul suffers from hydrocafelin or water on the brain, and didn't lose his eye sight until he was six-years-old. In June 1999, at the Potteries Marathon in Staffordshire, Paul became the first blind person to run 100 marathons.

"Yes, I think you need courage to run blind, or have your brains looked at," said Paul, who had drawn inspiration about running marathons while lying in hospital for five-and-a-half weeks with a broken leg. "This was back in 1982 just about the time when the London Marathon first started. I was too young to apply just then as I had only turned 18, but it was while I was in hospital that I decided a marathon was one of the things I wanted to do."

It wasn't until seven years later that Paul completed his first marathon, the London Marathon, guided round by a friend, Derek John, who had trained him for the event. Since then, Paul has not looked back. "Since I became a member of the 100 Club I really enjoy my running," he added. "There is such great camaraderie. I have some sight, but I need someone to run with me and guide me round. Mostly runners are very kind, but there are one or two who can be a little awkward."

Highlight for Paul was his 100th marathon which took place in Stoke when he ran the final 30 metres unaided to be greeted by a finish line full of runners. "It was a very memorable moment and the hairs on the back of my neck were standing up," he said. "It was an amazing moment."

A year earlier, I had trained for a couple of months with a blind runner who was hoping to compete in the Great South Run in Portsmouth, so I got some idea what it was like to pace someone without sight, choosing a path which was clear of obstacles. Sadly, my friend, Steve, failed to make the start line after getting injured. I would joke as we ran around Southampton Common about some of the attractive female joggers who were running past us. He always wanted a full description of what they looked like. Sadly, having fallen blind late in life, Steve's marriage also went down the pan when his wife had an affair. "You know what, I didn't even see it coming!"

Meanwhile, Paul, who runs up to 30 miles a week either with his club or on a treadmill and cross-trainer at home, has no idea how many blind runners there are in the UK. Most tend to run on the track, but fewer opt for the road. He said he enjoys running with a guide since they can chat and have a good time. He never runs on his own. The only downside is that he misses out on the scenery at some of the spectacular events.

He is hoping by the end of 2008 to have completed 200 marathons. "I don't know how long I will carry on running for. I thought I might give up after my 100th marathon but I didn't. I'm now aiming for my 200th marathon and I hope to get to 300. I might call it a day after that, but who knows."

I left Paul and his guides behind at the village of St Judes which provided the ten mile marker, before a gentle run-in to Ramsey and the finish in front of a good-sized crowd sat in the main stand. I felt good, I felt energised, and this was just the boost I needed.

51. St Levan 10km @ Penzance, Cornwall.

THIS year was full-on enough without outside distractions. However on the day I was driving to Cornwall I was weighing up the options of accepting a new job. I had been offered the chance to become editor of the Swindon Advertiser, a daily paper in Wiltshire and part of the same Newsquest group which I worked for as deputy editor with the Southern Daily Echo in Southampton. It was a tricky decision. I was quite content in Southampton but the chance to finally achieve my dream of becoming an editor had presented itself at my feet. Despite the upheaval it might cause, this was an opportunity which I couldn't pass up on.

So on the long drive to St Levan, I was weighing up the consequences and how I could take up the job. With my family based on the south coast, and having fought for many years to get the right package of social care for Ross, there was no way I was going to uproot them. Equally, Swindon is a 75 minute drive from Southampton and not commutable. What was I going to do? Take the job, of course!

In terms of the 80-event challenge, the St Levan 10km race was a major marker. In May, I had flown and then driven hundreds of miles to Cape Wrath at the north-west tip of Scotland to take part in the northernmost race in the British Isles. Now, on a humid August evening I was in Cornwall, three miles from Land's End for the most westerly, and the most southerly race in mainland UK. (I did race in Guernsey in April which technically lies further south!). So I set out from Southampton early on Friday morning for the long drive to the south-west. Fortunately the roads weren't too bad; just a few hold-ups when tractor drivers decided to use the main A-road to crawl along oblivious to the long tail-back behind them.

I reached Land's End in good time to take a break to visit the place which has caught people's imagination for thousands of years. The Romans described Land's End as "Bolerium", the seat of storms, and its old Cornish name is "Penn-an-Wlas" meaning end of the land. It is a location of stunning scenery and fabled views looking out towards the Scilly Isles from the 200ft high cliffs.

St Levan is a small village on a quiet country road just outside Land's End. This annual race is surprisingly popular among locals and holidaymakers; there was a fair sprinkling of running vests from around the country such as Penny Lane Striders from Merseyside, Keighley & Craven AC in Yorkshire, Bournville Harriers from Birmingham and East Antrim Harriers from Northern Ireland. The 10km race has been going since 1990, organised as part of the village's sports week. In 1999, the total eclipse of the sun put paid to the run because of fears that Cornwall would be gridlocked for days – in the end, the eclipse turned out to be an over-hyped non-event.

Come Friday evening, there was a buzz in St Levan as cars parked on the sports field, the announcer was trying to whip up some excitement, and the sale of Cornish pasties from inside the village hall was going well.

The sudden start on the main road outside the Methodist Chapel caught everyone by surprise as we set off past the duck pond at Polgigga and then a right hand through Trebehor. By the time we hit a long descent to the wonderfully named Bottoms, we were being caught by some of the fun runners who were fizzing past. One kid was wearing an iPod, unaware that his shouts of "excuse me, excuse me!" could be heard as far away as Penzance.

The first couple of miles along country lanes to Bosfranken Farm and Penrose were hilly and twisty, but made for challenging running. The second half of the race was a lot easier and pleasant. The weather was humid. Sadly, views over the sea were not existent as the course skirted inland, but there was great support as you re-entered St Levan and rounded off the 10km with a swift circuit around the sports field to the finish.

I was placed 71st from 181 runners in a time of 46 minutes 33 seconds. I honestly thought I had run a little faster, but with a race the following day and a 270-mile trip to get there, I was holding back a little.

52. Race The Train @ Twyn, North Wales.

IF you love running, then Race The Train is one of the must-do races. It is unique, it is challenging and it is fun, and after my first ever bash at this popular event, I know I will be back.

Race The Train takes place in the coastal town of Tywyn in mid-Wales, north of Aberystwyth, and this was the 24th staging of the multi-terrain run which is organised by the town's Rotary club. Every year, profits from the race are donated to charities.

Just down the road at Llanwrtyd Wells there is the annual Man versus Horse race over 22 miles and in 2004, Londoner Huw Lobb picked up the £25,000 prize when he beat his equine rival for the first time in the event's 25 year history. So the Welsh are used to putting on these madcap races.

In Tywyn, runners go head to head with a train which runs along the Talyllyn Railway. The steam train pulls out of Tywyn Wharf and heads up through the valley past Rhydyronen, Brynglas, Dolgoch Falls to Nant Gwernol, and then turns round before making the trip back along a route, much of which lies within the Snowdonia National Park.

The Talyllyn Railway is a narrow gauge line for steam locomotives which was opened in 1865 and was once a working line serving the slate mines in the valley. Many valleys in North and Mid Wales hosted narrow-gauge railways, which were cheaper to build through mountainous terrain than full-size railways.

The decline of quarrying and mining and the rise of the lorry forced many to close from the 1930s. The writing was on the wall for the Talyllyn Railway when its owner died in 1950, but a group of enthusiasts and engineers persuaded the owner's widow that they could keep the railway open, using volunteer labour. Today the railway attracts thousands of people every year for the ride from Tywyn along a beautiful green valley to Abergynolwyn and Nant Gwernol, close to Cader Idris. The railway still uses some of its original equipment, including a steam engine from 1864. The Talyllyn was the first railway in the world to be saved by volunteer labour.

And what of the race? Earlier in the day there were a 5 mile, 10km and junior races, but the biggie is the 14.75-miler which starts on a sports ground adjacent to Talyllyn Railway Wharf Station. It is superbly organised with a huge marquee stationed in the centre of the field offering food, seating and tables, along with protection from the elements.

The first mile and a bit out of Tywyn was gentle as runners headed through the town towards Brynglas. The race started at 2:05pm, the train left 20 minutes later. At Brynglas, we turned up a farm track to cross over the railway line which we traced all the way to Rhyd-yr-Onnen. Despite it being August, the weather was grey and overcast, though still humid. It was pretty clear early on once we stepped into the country that this was going to be a muddy race. The first short but stiff climb tested the multi-terrain footwear on a grassy hill.

Everyone had been warned to take it steady for the first half of the race because the second half would be even tougher. The rain began falling as the huge field of runners, who had come from all over the country, tackled the mixture of tracks and field and one stretch where you waded through a ford. It was mucky, it was dirty, it was a slog. You were picking your way along tracks trying to avoid the cowpats, plotting a path where the ground was firm. At times it was single file running as you had to be patient behind runners in front.

I ran most of the race with Stubbington Green Runner team-mate, Richard Simms, who had driven up to Mid-Wales with his family. I'd driven straight up to Wales from Cornwall, broken up with an overnight stay in Bristol. Richard and I took it in turns to lead, and set out at a gentle eight minute mile pace navigating our way over fields and rough pasture to Dolgoch, running through a car park, and then along an unmade track to some well-cultivated pasture which had been ploughed just the day before. It was soul-destroying trying to pick your way through the gloopy mud of this field which had been ploughed right up to the edge.

It was at this point that, seven miles into the race, that I saw the steam train for the first time, a trail of smoke spiralling into the sky. We could hear the whistle sounding several miles back, and then to our right the train came into view with supporters waving and cheering at us from the three carriages being pulled by the Victorian engine. It was hard to look up safely since we were wading through ankle high mud.

This was the turning point as we crossed a stream and then climbed steeply across the face of the hillside on narrow sheep tracks. This part of the race was a killer. You were running on a slight camber with one foot higher than another. It took all your concentration to keep your balance and footing. Take one wrong step on the muddy and sodden tracks and you could tumble 20 feet down the hillside. We were now following some of the well-worn tracks used for the 10km race in the morning which made conditions even more treacherous. Again it was single-file order for some of the way. Some of the climbs simply had to be walked up. We passed a stunning waterfall at Dolgoch at the 10-mile mark. By this time, Richard had moved some 50 metres ahead, a gap I was unable to close.

My legs were growing increasingly tired, I was thoroughly wet and the fact that I had run a 10km race in Cornwall the night before was beginning to tell. It was fairly evident that there was no way we were going to beat to train, even though Richard and I steadily moved our way past tiring runners over the last few miles.

You needed to complete the 14.75-mile race in around 1 hour 47 minutes. Ordinarily on a road, that would be extremely gettable, but amid the wild Welsh mountains with rain pouring and difficult conditions, only the top 10 per cent managed to beat the train. The only way I was going to beat the Talyllyn train on this August day was if there had been overrunning track repairs with a diversion via Clapham Junction. Still, I was pleased with my finish which was surprisingly strong. I dug in for the last few miles and crossed the finish line in 2 hours 9 minutes. That was a thoroughly satisfying race and enormously rewarding. It is not as hard as a marathon physically, but this is a mental test – and you have got to be mental if you think you can out run a train!

53. Battle of Sedgemoor 10km @ Langport, Somerset

SOMERSET is not only famous for cider, cheese and The Wurzels, but the fact that in 1685 the last pitched battle in England took place there.

The Battle of Sedgemoor was fought on July 6th, 1685, between troops of the rebel James Scott, the first Duke of Monmouth and James II. After landing at Lyme Regis in Dorset, the Duke led his untrained and ill-equipped troops on a night-time attack on the King's position near the delightfully-named village of Westonzoyland.

However the element of surprise was lost when a musket was accidentally fired and all hell broke loose as the Duke's ragged troop was defeated by the Royal Army. Monmouth escaped but was eventually captured to be taken to the Tower of London where, after several meaty blows with an axe, he was beheaded.

So it is against this background that every summer this historic event is marked by the Battle of Sedgemoor 10km road race held in the Somerset town of Langport.

Originally I had planned to head for the Lake District to take part in the historic Grasmere Games' guides races; a two-mile fell race which is more than 150 years old. The hotel had been booked, I had planned to take my children to Grasmere to enjoy some traditional pastimes such as sheep dog trials, dancing and wrestling. But the best laid plans went to pot when I realised that I wouldn't be able to get back in time to make the Eurotunnel train to Calais for a brief family holiday in Holland. So a trip to cider country beckoned instead.

And what a great race it was. I had picked up a painful blister from Race The Train a week earlier, and this was causing me a little discomfort around the country lanes of Somerset which, compared to mid-Wales, was a much gentler affair.

I decided to give my son Ross a run-out in his sport stroller. Either Ross had put on weight or I was getting unfit because pushing my 10-year-old around was tougher. There were only a few hills; one leading out of Langport and another in the countryside, plus a couple of slight inclines towards the end. It was also pretty hot and humid.

The reception you get from running with a sports buggy tends to be mixed. Many runners will encourage you as you draw up alongside, and inevitably marshals and spectators offer support on the way round. But there are some runners who are clearly cheesed off. You can tell by their body language and their silence that they were not happy to see a runner flying by pushing a young boy in a buggy. You can see them eyeing you up and thinking: "You're taking the mick, fella."

The race consisted of a loop around Langport running through the town to the finish. A kilometre from the end we were directed to come off the road and run on the pavement, under some scaffolding where a building was being repaired. I was running at full pelt winding up for a strong finish but totally misjudged the gap between the scaffolding poles and crashed into the metal frame. My buggy wouldn't fit. Two runners collided with me from behind. It was a Keystone Cops moment. Fortunately the scaffolding held firm while the runners behind were only slightly winded by the emergency stop.

Ross was, as usual, pretty non-plussed by the drama as I quickly navigated the buggy briefly onto the road, around the scaffolding and back on the pavement. We ran just under 51 minutes for 10km and at the finish picked up one of the best mementoes of the year so far – a lush, green embroidered towel. What a great idea from Langport Runners and it made a change from the t-shirts and medals which were now clogging up my bedroom drawer.

"Marathon running is like cutting youself unexpectedly. You dip into the pain so gradually that the damage is done before you are aware of it. Unfortunately, when the awareness comes, it is excruciating."

SEP2007

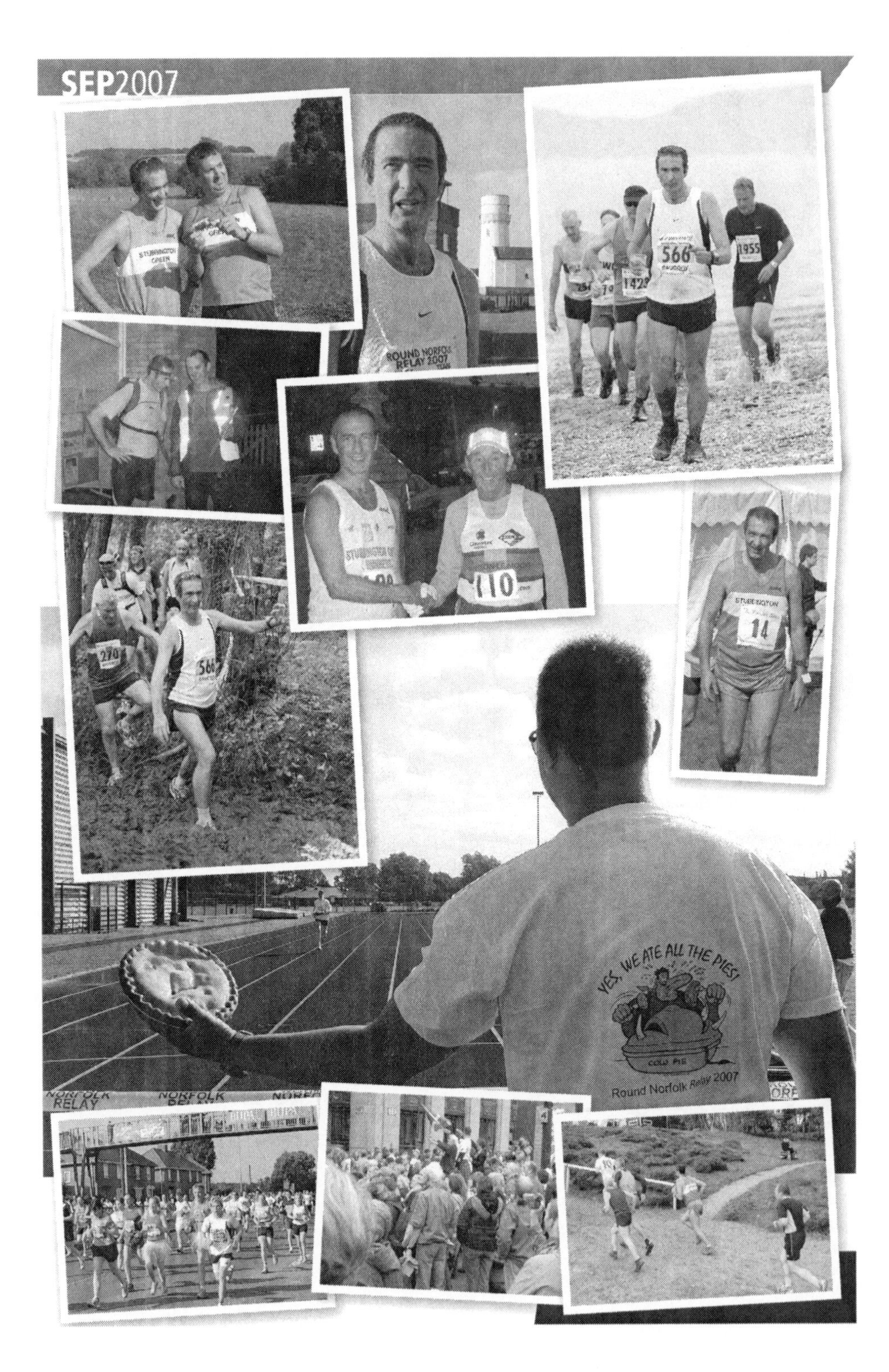

STUBBINGTON GREEN
ROUND NORFOLK RELAY 2007
566
1955
110
14
270
YES, WE ATE ALL THE PIES!
COW PIE
Round Norfolk Relay 2007
NORFOLK RELAY

SEPTEMBER

54. Braemar Highland Games @ Braemar Castle, Royal Deeside, Scotland.

SNUBBED by the Queen – can you believe it? While Her Majesty was tucking into lunch at nearby Balmoral Castle, the royals' summer retreat, I was running my heart out at the Braemar Highland Gathering. Just as she was deciding whether to opt for strawberry tartlet or plain cheese and biscuits, I was slogging my guts out climbing a lung-busting 2,800ft mountain perched on the edge of the Cairngorms.

Then half an hour later, 17,000 spectators sat in ringside seats or on the grassy bowl surrounding the main arena greeted the arrival of the exhausted returning runners with thunderous applause. With a searing sprint over the soft turf, I crossed the finish line in front of the patron's box feeling physically sick. I looked up expecting to receive royal approval for my stoic effort, only for the Queen's seat and those in the royal party to be occupied by the children of some Highland bigwig playing scissors, stone and paper! What a downer!!

I was later told by a police officer that Her Majesty, who is patron of the Braemar Royal Highland Society, would not be turning up to the gathering for another hour when the massed piped bands parade would take place in the arena. Hopefully she would have digested her hearty lunch. By then I'd had enough of the wall-to-wall bagpipes and decided to take my leave with my dad who was in tow.

The Braemar Highland Gathering is something else. Here is a tradition going back thousands of years when various Highland Games were staged under the sponsorship of kings and clan chiefs. They were an ideal recruiting agency. For example, winners of the athletic races made excellent couriers and the strongest men served as fine bodyguards – or wine bottle openers! Athletes, wrestlers, dancers and pipers were trained by the chiefs for the glory which their prowess reflected on their masters. I'm not sure what job I would have got based on my athletic prowess – plate scrubber maybe?!

The Braemar Gathering on Royal Deeside has been held since the 18th century. It is a magnificent occasion, brimming with pomp, ceremony and tradition, set against a jaw-dropping mountainous backdrop. Dancers, pipers, strongmen and athletes take to the stage for an occasion which is quaint, dignified and represents a true slice of Scottish life.

My bit-part was participating in the Morrone Hill Race. As we assembled for the start in the main arena I looked at the hardened fell-runners around me feeling seriously out of my depth. Their craggy worn faces and elephant skin bodies carried the scars and stories of the hard men of the fells; those for whom injury was an incidental occupation. I was cruising for a bruising, and this was going to hurt. However before I could nurse any further doubts we were off and making our way towards the Five Cairns.

The 3.3-mile run featured a back-breaking 1,000ft climb initially through boggy peat, across heather and then up a rock-strewn path which wound its way to the summit at a ridiculous angle. With every stride my hamstring ached as a ribbon of runners stretched upwards to the skyline. It was a 25 minute gut-wrenching, hamstring-hurting, back-breaking climb to the summit.

At the top we were handed wrist bands to indicate we had reached the summit. There was no cheating here. You couldn't chicken out by hiding half way up the mountain, and then filtering in among the runners hurtling down to the finish.

"Enjoy the view when you get to the summit," one of the experienced local runners advised me beforehand. "It'll make the climb worth it." The view was impressive, staring at miles upon miles of the craggy Cairngorms. Down below lay the multi-coloured specks of cars parked neatly in rows behind the small but smart Princess Royal and Duke of Fife Memorial Park which hosts the Braemar Gathering.

There wasn't much time to enjoy the spectacle. The task ahead was to throw myself off the summit, running as fast as I dared hugging a terrifying slope which stretched out below. Careering downhill at a suicidal speed, my feet bouncing off the lush mountainside heather which provided a soft purple carpet, I was, to use a technical running term, bricking it big time!

The feeling of heather underfoot was bizarre; soft and springy. The smooth cushion surface fooled you into a false sense of security because then, just as I was coping with an even pace, disaster struck. My right foot reached out for terra firma and met with thin air as my foot then disappeared down a hole.

Suddenly my body hurtled face forward. I was scared. Nine months of racing was about to be shattered as my foot became caught in a crag with the rest of my 12 stone body crashing to the ground like a felled tree. It happened so slowly. I was in freefall, pushing my arms out to break the fall, and then impact. I waited for the crack in my leg, I braced myself for my brain to register the searing pain, I anticipated the awful reality that after nine months of toil my bid to run around the British Isles in 80 races was over - thwarted by a broken ankle on a Scottish hillside.

But then nothing. Nothing happened. Nothing at all. No pain, no crack. I gingerly lifted myself off the bed of soft heather still expecting the pain to sneak up on me. But despite being winded and my ankle throbbing with slight discomfort, I was fine. The number pinned to my vest was flapping in the gentle breeze so I took half a minute to adjust, get my breath again, and set off again.

Soon I was back into my stride as the heather carpet was swapped for a narrow rocky path. Other runners chose more adventurous downhill routes, but I was playing this one conservatively. I chased down those runners ahead. I had come into the race worried I wouldn't be competitive, up against seasoned fell runners who were small, sinewy and tough. Guys who would make mincemeat of the Sassenach and where the course record, set in 1984, stands at an amazing 24 minutes 28 seconds set by Mick Hawkins from Grassington in North Yorkshire. However I surprised myself by more than holding my own; steady uphill and then, despite the tumble, pushing on strongly downhill.

The downhill leg took less than 15 minutes as we were ushered through gates towards the main arena. There, a crowd warmly greeted the runners for a final circuit on the grass turf.

Around us were highland dancers performing their traditional reels, muscle-bound Adonis-type creatures tossing the caber in their kilts, and a Highland marching band was playing a stirring tune on the bagpipes. The applause was uplifting as we came into the arena. This was a hair on the back of your neck moment. It was a long 300-metre finish around the edge of the arena. I put on a sprint passing two runners on the way.

I had survived yet not disgraced myself. A time of 41 minutes for the three-and-half mile run sounds slow, but believe me that was a pig of a hill to run up. More than that, I was delighted to have escaped injury-free from a fall which I believed would put an end to the year-long adventure. Fifty four races down, just 26 to go....such a shame Her Majesty missed it!

55. freshnlo Great Scottish Run @ Glasgow

A LITTLE less than 24 hours after surviving the Morrone Hill Race at Braemar I was driving along the M8 to Glasgow. My dad and I had spent the night in a cheap and tatty motel at Glenrothes on an industrial estate, our rest disturbed by a couple next door playing a modern version of the hokey-cokey – their exuberant noises through the thin walls just didn't sit right while watching Match of the Day with Gary Lineker and Alan Hansen blathering away.

The contrast of the past 24 hours couldn't have been greater. The rural spectacular of Royal Deeside was being compared to the sprawling metropolis of Scotland's second city. The quaintness of the Braemar Royal Highland Gathering was set head-to-head with a modern day race around Glasgow for the 26th edition of the freshnlo Great Scottish Run.

Driving to the edge of Glasgow, we took advantage of a park and ride on the Glasgow underground which was free to all runners. The train took us to George Square in the heart of the city beside the towering statue of Sir Walter Scott which was fronted by the impressive-looking City Chambers. The Square was buzzing with thousands of runners and spectators, enlivened by non-stop commentary to whip up an atmosphere. Even a sprightly-looking Sir Jimmy Saville was there to wave off runners in both the 10km and half marathon races.

Each race had four separate starts to avoid overcrowding. With runners wearing timing chips held by velcro strips strapped around their ankles, it meant you got an accurate finish time no matter what time you crossed the start line.

The pre-race set-up was magnificent, the weather was good; dry, but not too hot, and I was ready to race. But come half marathon race time at 10am, what a disappointment. The Great Scottish Run was one of the drabbest of races of the year – the anti-climax felt greater because I had expected better.

Glasgow doesn't set the world alight with its architecture, definitely not on the race route. We ran across Kingston Bridge, along grim streets, past dreary buildings in dire need of a lick of paint and along roads which were sparsely populated with spectators. Was this Stoke-on-Trent revisited?

The atmosphere around the course was downbeat and dead; this from a city which later that year would win the bid to host the Commonwealth Games in 2014. We ran through Bellahouston Park and then Pollok Country Park which offered some green relief from the inner city eyesores, before the final five miles on an uninspiring course towards the finish at Glasgow Green.

It was tough to run two races in two days, so after Braemar my legs were feeling very heavy. Luckily, just as we were crossing the River Clyde for a second time about a mile from the end, I spotted a familiar face in Syd Gallacher, deputy headmaster of a school in Campbelltown on the Mull of Kintyre. We had run together last May at the Mull of Kintyre Half Marathon. Back then I had pulled Syd round to a fast time, so on this occasion I was relieved that he could to return the favour.

Syd was brilliant. Just as I was faltering, he helped me with some well chosen words of encouragement to push on towards the finish on Glasgow Green. I crossed the line in just over 1 hour 39 minutes which was surprisingly slow since I had believed I was on for a 1 hour 36 minute half marathon. I then looked at my Garmin watch which measures the route which read the distance as 13.42 miles, instead of 13.1. It didn't matter. I had finished, but I think I'll give Glasgow a miss in the future.

56. Test Way Relay @ Stockbridge

THE Test Way Relay follows some of the most picturesque countryside in Hampshire. It traces a route from Inkpen Beacon, just over the border in Berkshire, to Eling near Southampton.

The River Test, threading its way along the length of Test Valley, is known the world over for the excellence of its fishing. Flowing through the chalk downland in the north, past the market town of Andover, and on to historic Stockbridge, the river widens and deepens as it flows south before meeting Southampton Water.

For walkers, and more especially runners, the Test Way footpath is not the easiest to follow, crossing fields, passing through woodland, and running alongside the riverbank skirting expensive million pound homes.

The Test Way Relay is a nine-stage relay with the ladies and mixed teams setting off on the 44-mile race at 10.30am, the men's teams go an hour later. This year was the 22nd running of the race, which was organised by Hardley Runners, who are based in the New Forest.

It was cold and a little nippy for the morning start, but by midday the weather had turned hot and humid. For once, it was great to be running with team-mates as part of a relay squad, albeit I was chosen to run for Stubbington Green Runners' slowest team on a 5.74-mile sixth leg from Stockbridge to Mottisfont.

By the time I took the handover at about 3pm, our team was one but last! I set off with no-one to chase, and no-one chasing me. The sixth leg was a simple one, heading from Stockbridge in the heart of the Test Valley on a straight four-mile stretch down a track. We crossed over a bridge by a jaw-droppingly expensive house which sits on the banks of the river and then headed for an uphill finish just outside Mottisfont Abbey - a 12th-century Augustinian priory.

I began at a pretty swift pace early on, but without anyone alongside and only the occasional passing cyclist for company, I became easily distracted. My mind wandered and my pace slowed. I was mindful I had a big race the following day so I tried to run conservatively.

The finish beckoned as a throng of people gathered at the top of the hill for the handover to the next green-vested Stubbington colleague. Our team finished one from last, but then someone had to!

57. The Grizzly @ Seaton, Devon

EARLIER this year, I ran the 26.2-miles of the London Marathon on a sweltering hot day in just under three-and-a-half hours.

Five months on I waddled across the finish line of The Grizzly on Devon's south coast having taken just under three-and-three-quarter hours to run a measly 19.7 miles. Guess which one was harder?

The title of this year's torture was Armageddon Now Here – a 2007 Grizzly Asylum of Running Production - an appropriate sub-text for the soul-destroying hardship which lay ahead, which only someone a few cards short of a full deck would take on!

This year's race was originally shipwrecked because of the container vessel MSC Napoli which spectacularly beached itself just off Branscombe Bay in January, prompting a flurry of scavengers to rifle through the cargo which had washed up on the beach

So Armageddon was delayed for six months. Instead of being staged on a windswept and damp March day, the tidy town of Seaton was bathed in sunshine for the September start. It was definitely sunglasses weather. Fortunately, the skies clouded over later in the morning, but still conditions were humid.

I was feeling decidedly uncertain and a wee bit worried about this race. I had left the trail shoes in my car and gone for lighter road wear. I've tended to get nasty blisters from trail shoes when running in excess of 10 miles, so I sacrificed tread for comfort. It was a gamble, and fortunately the choice of footwear proved to be the right one.

The race itself was a veritable pot-pourri of running. We began the race on the Esplanade in Seaton, setting out on a tricky half-mile stretch along the shingle, looping back towards the start line and then heading out of Seaton up the first hill. It was a stiff opening climb towards the cliff top which set the benchmark for the toughest of races as the field of almost 1,000 runners trailed through the pretty countryside.

A week ago in Glasgow, the atmosphere for a big city half marathon had been characterless and charmless. Here in the rural west country, there was a fantastic feelgood factor. Musicians including a bagpiper, folk musicians, drummers and even a fella playing a didgeredoo, lined the route, along with small knots of spectators who were handing out sweets and drinks. The Axe

Valley Runners' marshals were cheerful and smiling; it was this winning combination which helped to mask the pain of the race.

The passing scenery was spectacular – but it was scenery with a sting! The stricken shell of the Napoli lay off the coast as we ran over the cliff top down steep grassy paths and up twisting, testing climbs. The gradients soon became so severe that we were reduced to walking up the hills.

If that opening was the appetiser, then the main course was tough to stomach. The musical strains of a bagpiper heralded the first of the bogs almost knee deep in glutinous mud. More hazards were to follow. We crossed streams, pulled our way up one grassy hill which was close to vertical as could be. It was hard and relentless, and the pace was inevitably slow.

The miles ticked by slowly, the tactic was to survive by conserving energy on the uphill sections and then pushing on the downhills. Ten, 11, 12 and 13 miles passed. Soon the calves were cramping, the hamstring tightening. Runners around me were hurting too, stopping on the paths trying to rid their bodies of aches as lactic acid, like a poison in the body, built up in their legs. The Grizzly takes no prisoners and accepts no passengers.

Fourteen, 15, 16 and 17 miles followed as the course headed up horrendous hills and down dales through the villages of Bramscombe and Beer. The crowds continued to be superbly enthusiastic. I bagged a handful of jelly babies and Licorice All Sorts as we trekked across Branscombe Beach before stepping up the infamous Stairway To Heaven and over to the final cliff looking down to Seaton.

I couldn't wait for the race finish. I looked at my watch. I had been running longer than the London Marathon and seven miles shorter. The final assault was one last short beach run to the finish at Seaton Esplanade. Never before has a finish been so warmly received. Never before have I felt so knackered.

Firemen from the Dorset Fire Brigade were there to hose down our mud-strewn shoes and legs with seawater. There was a seawater shower on hand for good measure. The Grizzly was hard, it was tough, but boy did I feel a huge sense of achievement.

58. Round Norfolk Relay @ King's Lynn to Hunstanton.

SIX o'clock on a crisp autumn morning looking out over The Wash where a small fishing boat was gliding along the silky smooth waters – can there really be a better time to run? Dawn was breaking on the west Norfolk coastline, the sky above was a silvery blue waiting for the sun's radiance to break through.

Along the coastal path an ethereal mist hung over the fields. There was no-one about, the silence was occasionally broken by the early morning ornithological choir.

This was the first leg of the 193-mile Round Norfolk Relay, a 16-mile opener between King's Lynn and Hunstanton. I have never considered myself much of a pie eater - steak and kidney maybe, the occasional pork pie, but I'm not what you call lardy! So I was honoured to be inducted into the running team with the fabulous name of Yes We Ate All The Pies for this year's relay.

YWAATP are a group of friends from Lowestoft and London who have known each other for donkeys' years through school and a diving club.

Eighteen months ago the idea was sewn that they should get together for a weekend of running; gathering on a Saturday evening for a pre-race meal, run a half marathon on the Sunday, and then reconvene for a boozy, post-race celebration.

The half marathon was soon ditched in favour of the relay and in 2006, YWAATP took their bow in this challenging event. Twelve months ago there were only three slower teams than the pie-eaters from the 45 starters. "At least with our unusual name people know from the outset what we are all about," explained Andy, a 36-year-old Royal Navy weapon technician. "They know we are here to run, but we're here to have fun as well."

Andy, dressed in a wonderful Belicia Beacon orange outfit, was my cycling guide on the first leg; the dawn-breaking opener to sunny Hunny. As one of the slowest teams, we had been given the earliest start among seven other snails which meant a 6am off; many runners had slept overnight at the local leisure centre so as not to miss the beginning of the race. The hares wouldn't be leaving the Lynnsport leisure centre for two or three more hours. But for me this early start wasn't a punishment, this was a reward for running at the most perfect time of the day.

Dawn was breaking as we set off at six o' clock. Two guys went scorching off into the lead, never to be seen again. I was running very respectable seven minute miles so how slow were these guys?

Andy was brilliant. He provided great conversation, encouragement and drinks of water along the way. We were alone for most of the opening miles heading out of King's Lynn to Castle Rising, and then on forest roads bordering the Sandringham estate – my second close encounter with royalty in a month.

Our route cut in towards the coast, through the delightful village of Wolferton where the old railway station stood, complete with white gates and platform which someone had converted in a home. It was here that Andy could cycle no further because I was about to head onto a shingly beach. He turned round to meet up with his partner and fellow runner Heidi, a 35-

year-old customs officer, who was following in a car behind. Andy chucked his bike in the boot and drove off to the next crossing point. They were also joined in the car by Rebecca, a 25-year-old charity fund-raiser with a lovely lilting Welsh accent, who I would be handing over to at the end of this first leg.

The route along the coast was hard since the sand and shingle surface dragged at my ankles, pulling my calfs and pounding the hamstrings. It was like running in treacle, fortunately the spectacular scenery provided a wonderful anesthetic to the pain.

Soon the sky was lifting from a silver grey to blue, the sea was silky smooth and serene, and a low mist hung over the coastal plain graced by a chorus of birds.

It was a very pleasurable experience. The route was well marked so there were few problems along the way and the laminated map I carried was surplus to requirements. From time to time I met the odd birdwatcher resting on a gate with binoculars trained towards the marshes, plus the occasional walker.

The sereneness of the run was shattered half way through by a sudden call of nature. I usually take Immodium for long runs which constipates the bowels, but I had forgotten to pack the tablets on the drive to East Anglia. I'd felt uncomfortable early on but there was no way I was going to dash into the bushes with Andy around. So I waited until he had rejoined Heidi and Rebecca before having a quick constitutional, apologised to a nearby flock of ducks for the sewage smell, and continued on my way!

Relief was at hand, no not for the bottom, but for my weary feet when, after passing Heacham and Snettisham, the route returned to hard-standing and solid Tarmac along the promenade. The seaside town of Hunstanton hove into view. Beach huts and small wooden seaside shelters had closed down for the winter, as had the fairground. Now I was on the run-in for home.

The final stretch involved a series of dog legs up a path by the cliffs, and then a sprint towards the lighthouse for the end of my leg. There was Rebecca ready and waiting for me to hand over the hollow metal baton, which made for a great pan-pipe instrument along some of the windier stretches of the coast!

I handed over in third place in a time of 2 hours 9 minutes for the 16.38 mile run. My hamstring was pulling quite a bit, still feeling the effects of the Grizzly the previous week. It concerned me so much so that I abandoned plans to compete in the Experian Robin Hood Half Marathon in Nottingham the following day.

Once recovered from the run, Heidi was waiting in the car with Joe, who had driven straight to Hunstanton and was armed with a bagful of pies. We jumped into the car and set off in pursuit of Rebecca. I stayed with the team for the next couple of stages which took runners to Burnham Overy and Wells where I met more members of the mad YWAATP team.

The following day the team eventually crossed the finish line without too many mishaps in a time of 28 hours 50 minutes and 8 seconds - some 21 minutes faster than 2006, but still the third slowest of all the teams. It didn't matter. The pie-eaters had a blast.

59. Sleepwalker Midnight Marathon @ Talybont on Usk, South Wales

IT'S fast approaching midnight and I'm 2,000 feet up a mountain in the heart of the Brecon Beacons. It's windy, though fortunately the temperature is not too cool. Ahead of me, half a mile distant, I can pick out a pair of headlights shining from a jeep.

I've already been running for two hours and my body is beginning to ache. The light from my head-torch tries to map out the rocky path ahead, but with tired legs I am no longer picking up my feet.

Suddenly my legs are taken away from me. I trip on rocks and with a heavy rucksack weighted on my back this adds to the downward momentum. I hardly have time to break the fall by putting out my arms, instead I land slightly on my side taking the impact on my elbows and cheek. I let out a cry in the dark as I hit the deck, more out of annoyance than pain.

All is still. My heart is racing. It is the autumn equinox and there is a three-quarter moon above. Stars resonate faint traces of light, the wind blows across the desolate land. I'm hurt. I can feel the trickle of blood on my elbows and on my knees. My jaw aches too. It's no time to wimp out or feel sorry for myself, all I can do is to pick myself up and carry on.

Five minutes later I reach the Jeep. It's the mountain rescue team who are keeping tabs on runners competing in the Sleepwalker Mountain Marathon.

"What's your number, mate?" asks one.

"Six."

"You're doing fine. Half way there, only 10 miles to go."

I reply: "You don't know where the nearest KFC is, do you?" The guys from the mountain rescue laugh, and climb back into their Jeep while I push on.

This is running at its most stupid. The thought of taking on one of the most treacherous mountain ranges in Britain at night sounds challenging and mad, but it is very unfulfilling. The organisers' pre-race literature describes the route like a holiday brochure…."a wonderful running route in the Brecon Beacons National Park taking in parts of the Vaughan Way, Beacons Way and Taff Trail" …."the route undulates through mature forest with, weather permitting, tantalizing moonlit views over the reservoir and hills beyond before climbing up through the Brecon Beacons on a 2,000 year-old Roman Road." ..."the route crosses a rugged pass between the high summits".

Moonlit views? I couldn't see a sausage! It was a bit like lying on a beach in Barbados which was shrouded in fog, or driving through the Alps in a fierce snow blizzard – it may be nice outside, but you can't see a thing.

According to organiser Duncan Clark, the idea for the Sleepwalker came after reminiscing about the night races he used to do as a teenager at the King Henry VIII School in Coventry. "Ted Norrish, who set up the Octavian Droobers orienteering club, used to organise an annual night orienteering event of about 16 miles, normally in Shropshire around the Long Mynd, Stiperstones or sometimes up in the White Peak," he explained.

"In those days it was quite permissible to allow pairs of 14 year olds to run on their own in these events - sadly legislation has put an end to so much adventure for youngsters, which is why I had to stipulate an 18 years old age limit on the Sleepwalker.

"Realisingthattheredweren'tmany,ifany,nightracesbeingorganised,Idecided I had better do something about it – that's right- if you want something doing....

"Choosing the Brecon Beacons as a venue was pretty easy, as the terrain is so fantastic and well suited to running events - also I've been spending a fair amount of time down there working with Bob Spour of the SASsurvival Company, so it seemed logical that we would hold it here.

"The course is aimed at anyone who is up for a bit of an adventure, as well as experienced trail racers and anyone who fancies another training opportunity in the Brecon Beacons."

Part of the Brecon Beacons' splendour is the spectacular views, the amazing countryside, the wonderment of nature. Occasionally you could pick out the orange glow of street lights from a village below, but this trail race was just one dull run. When you are running with a head torch and can barely see a few feet in front of you hour after hour, believe me, it becomes monotonous.

About 50 runners set out from the village hall at Talybont-on-Usk at 9pm. This was the date of the Autumn Equinox. Beforehand, we each had our kit checked to ensure we were wearing trail shoes, carrying a head torch with spare batteries, as well as packing waterproofs, maps, survival bag, whistle, and some spare clothing, including hat and gloves.

Messages from the race organisers were mixed. We had been warned this was not a map-reading exercise – basic map reading required, no compass necessary - but then at the pre-race briefing it became clear knowing your way round the various map markings was going to be fundamental and I was worried. My map reading is very basic.

As we set off by the canal in this quiet Welsh village, a couple of runners set off to the front. I led the second group, little did they know I had no idea where we were going. I fell several times early on as we worked our way along forest paths and trails. There was little conversation, the stillness of the night was only disturbed by the rhythmic sound of our feet. With a head torch as a guide in the pitch dark, it was hard to pick the way ahead as stumbling feet inevitably caught on rocks or tripped over branches strewn across the path.

Soon our group was whittled down to three. We passed a couple of checkpoints manned by mountain rescue teams who counted us all by. I wasn't enjoying the race one bit. Whereas in daylight you could enjoy the spectacular scenery and bask in the sheer wilderness, in the dark it was claustrophobic and dull.

We climbed 2,000 feet to the highest point of the route, a climb I made by myself having felt the need to push on to chase a couple of runners whose lights I could see in the distance. The descent was as equally treacherous as the ascent. Hour after hour we ran, and finally, chasing the two runners ahead of me, we arrived at the canal path for home.

The falls had damaged my Garmin watch which measured the race distance. As I became detached from the two pacers for this final stint, my mind became fatigued. I was becoming disorientated and my body distressed with the pain. I was hurting. My whole body ached and hurt, really hurt.

But without warning and believing I had a further two miles to run because of the damaged Garmin, I arrived at a bridge where Liz had been standing. She called out to me. Her voice was music to my ears as she directed me off the canal path for the short run in to the village hall where, exhausted, I crossed the line - well, there was a guy with a clipboard standing outside the hall who asked me my race number. I had finished 11th from 50 runners in a time of 3 hours 54 minutes.

Afterwards, the other survivors spoke in glowing tones about the race. Conversations focused on how taxing the challenge was, revelling in the camaraderie, describing how exhilarating it was to complete the midnight marathon. I could only be thankful I had finished and more through luck than judgment had got my way round the Brecon Beacons safely. Fortunately the weather had been kind. God forbid had there been rain or mist up on the hills.

For some, the race was going to take up to ten hours. I just wanted to get to the B&B and go to bed. This was, without doubt, my most painful and dullest race of the year.

60. Ron Hill Birthday 5km @ Littleborough near Rochdale

RON Hill is probably the greatest runner this country has ever had. Three Olympic Games, a European Championship gold medal, setting a world marathon best as well as countless British records, understate what a colossus King Ron was during the 1960s and 1970s.

He was running the sort of marathon times 30 years ago which few British men can achieve today. Ron celebrated his 69th birthday in September 2007 when I caught up with him at his home in Hyde, just outside of Manchester.

He still looked as thin and trim as ever. Sporting a baseball cap, jeans and a sports top, we chatted for over an hour about those halcyon days of running comparing that sepia era with the sport today.

Remarkably, Ron has continued an unbroken streak of running every day since 1964. Come fair weather or foul, he has been out there, sometimes running twice a day.

When we met on that sunny September afternoon, Ron talked about his globetrotting mission to run in 100 countries by the time of his 70th birthday in 2008. Recent trips to Ecuador and back-to-back runs in Argentina and Uruguay had taken that number up into the nineties. He was planning a trip later in the year to Montenegro which would boost the figure to 96. "I'm not interested in running at either the North Pole or South Pole – I don't like cold weather!

"I've done it with times and records, this is my way of keeping myself interested in my running," explained Ron.

And according to the diligent diary Ron has kept since September 3rd, 1956, he had, by his reckoning taken part in 2,300 races running over 150,000 miles – he would like to reach the magical 200,000 before being forced to hang up his running shoes.

"That's six times around the world," explained Ron. "I ran my 100,000th around the ground at Old Trafford in 1985. I remember the West Ham fans booed me that day!

"I didn't really start running until I was 14 or 15 in my last year at school. I have run every single day since 1964, after I had a terrible Olympic Games in Tokyo. I told myself I had to be more serious about my training and then I was running twice a day most days.

"It was two to three years later when I actually realised I had not missed a day's running – I was running 90 to 100 miles a week in the early days, and then in the 70s around 140 miles a week. A lot of the entries from my diary in 1967 read 'shattered' and 'very tired', but I have kept going.

"In 1993 I broke my sternum in a head-on crash, but I had run that morning and, as I was released from hospital the next day, I was able to run a mile at night even though it was agony. I have not missed a day."

It was a pleasure and an honour to chat to Ron, who has a passion for running and his sport. His was a generation when athletics made the back pages and runners were heroes. Today, Ron laments how the sport hardly generates any media coverage at all.

Does he look on the current crop of paid athletes with envy? Of course he does, but he nurtures no regrets about what he achieved, the races he ran or the records he set. "I think I have only had one massage in my life," admitted Ron, who after studying for a PhD in textile chemistry, would run to work each day to the research company in Droylsden.

"You know I never had a day off work. I would sometimes get sore throats or a chest infection, and possibly a head cold, but I would shrug it off. I would blame the kids, but now I realise that it was probably down to over-training then. But illness never stopped me.

"I used to drive to work on Monday and then run the seven miles there and back until Friday when I drove home for the weekend. I used to add bits and pieces if I needed to increase my mileage. I was at home at 6pm with my wife and my family, so with my run finished I didn't get too much pressure at home."

This from a man who typically at weekends would go for a five-mile run on the Saturday morning, race on Saturday afternoon, and opt for a stretch on Sunday with a gentle 21-mile run-out.

This from a man who describes running as "not rocket science, a sport which people tend to over-complicate".

And this from a man whose childhood hero was the post-War comic character Alf Tupper, who had to work hard for success since he faced a lot of obstacles in life. Alf Tupper was a fictional, working class, hard as nails runner, whose adventures under the title "Tough of the Track", appeared first in the "Rover" and then the "Victor" comics, over a 40 year period. Alf's most endearing characteristic was his love of fish and chips, not perhaps the kind of diet enjoyed by today's professional athletes!

During his athletics career, Ron brought out his own brand of sports clothing. On my way to the interview, I called into a sports shop in Hyde near his home to buy a Ron Hill sports top for the big man to sign, only to be told that he is no longer involved with the company and now has his own Hilly Clothing brand. Never mind the embarrassing oversight, Ron was still happy to sign the top which was later put to good use in a charity raffle.

But the great man was a pioneer of the day, conditioning himself in a way other athletes were not. He was aware of the glycogen levels in your body, the need to keep close tabs on diet, even wearing the right clothing for races.

"I more or less had to give up work as they wanted me to use my holidays to run for Great Britain," added Ron, who had his run-in with the selectors during an era when the Amateur Athletics Association really was amateur, and the tough working lad from the north seemed to suffer from the idiosyncrasies of the selectors.

"I think I would have had more success in the big championships if the selectors had had more faith in me. I always seemed to be fighting the system.

"The highlight was running two hours 9 minutes to win the Commonwealth Games marathon in Edinburgh in 1970 and breaking the Boston marathon course record when I ran two hours 10 minutes. I also enjoyed winning the European Championships in 1969 when it was run from Marathon to Athens, the site of the original marathon.

"The tar was melting and it was hilly. I didn't get to the front until there was one kilometre to go, so it was very dramatic. No-one expected me to win it."

Ron's biggest disappointment was failing to win a medal at the 1972 Olympics where he was one of the favourites for the marathon gold. "I did altitude training and went on a special diet, but I did it all too severely – you just didn't know in those days. I ended up finishing sixth. It all back-fired, but I know I did my best."

The big man has suffered various niggling injuries in recent years, but said that he intends to scale back his running after his 70th birthday.

I joined Ron later in the evening for a special birthday race which is held every year in his honour at Littleborough, just up the road near Rochdale.

It's a 5km race, organised by Ron's friend Andy O'Sullivan who I had met back at Freckleton in Lancashire that summer. Race headquarters was the Falcon Inn in the town.

Well over 100 runners turned up for the run which started at the unusual time of 6.45pm with Andy bellowing through his megaphone for runners to get to the start on time.

After the recent long runs, it was a pleasure to enjoy a shorter run which started at Littleborough taking runners through the streets and along a lane to Hollingworth Lake, before heading back into town and a finish by the railway station.

I settled in for a nice gentle run and clocked 22min 42sec for the distance a few minutes ahead of Ron, who in his prime ran 14 minutes for the distance.

Not that Ron was bothered. He is a legend, and long may he continue running.

61. BUPA Great North Run @ Newcastle, Tyneside.

IT was cold, bloody cold when I arrived in Newcastle for the start of the BUPA Great North Run. Mind you, it was 7.30am, more than three hours before race time. Yellow-bibbed marshals lined the carriageway, the public announcer was going through his "two-two, one-two" routine over the microphone, and there were just a few runners milling about.

You could see the breath in front of your face and for the first time this autumn, it was woolly hat weather.

How ironic that some five hours later, by the time runners were sweeping into the finish in South Shields, the weather boasted blazing sunshine as temperature was to play a major factor for the 13-mile race.

This was my first Great North. I had taken part in a few Great South Runs in Portsmouth but by comparison, this was a biggie. It's even bigger than the London Marathon with an estimated 50,000 runners taking part in the north-eastern jamboree.

The atmosphere is bigger and better too. With the marathon, there is tremendous nervous energy about the place with everyone apprehensive about the challenge which lies ahead. You're unsettled and it is hard to really enjoy the build-up or atmosphere around you. Your mind is so focused on the pain which is lurking around the corner. Running a half marathon is still a considerable feat of endurance but eminently more gettable.

Runners were in a more jocular and relaxed mood pre-race. I caught a park and ride bus from near Durham University where I had stayed the night. The bus arrived absurdly early in Newcastle for the start, so all I could do to kill the time was to put a running jacket down on the wet grass by a tree to park my bum, clip on my Ipod and read a newspaper for a few hours.

When race time arrived, I had a numb bum, had a drink and something to eat, put in a few stretches before ambling to the pen where I was placed. The organisers had wisely graded the pens according to predicted time, so the whippets were at the front, and the slower ones at the back. After all, there are few sports where mere mortals are able to rub shoulders with the greats, but running is one of them. So I, and the rest of the 50,000 throng, from club runners, to joggers and charity entries were able to run along the same Newcastle streets as Paula Radcliffe and those seriously fast Kenyans.

Not that I saw much of Paula, other than on a huge television screen which towered over the main carriageway of the A167 by the start at Spital

Tongues. She, along with the rest if the elite ladies' field, started half an hour ahead of the rest of us – any excuse to get in the showers first!

We were lined up on both sides of the carriageway in sections which were colour-coded according to our predicted times. The line of thousands upon thousands of runners stretched back and back past a row of double decker buses which would be transporting our bags to the finish line in South Shields.

One comedian managed to get to the front of the main race. As we heard the starter's gun plus the pounding music to herald the start of the BUPA Great North Run, we looked up on the TV screens to catch the BBC pictures being beamed from an overhead helicopter. Those around us laughed and applauded at the Linford Christie-like interloper who enjoyed his brief moment of front-running glory with a 100-metre sprint ahead of the elite gazelles.

The Great North Run is truly a running carnival. Where else can you witness so many bands playing along a race route, or for the event to be graced by a fly-past of the Red Arrows and a World War Two bomber?

That great Geordie ambassador, Brendan Foster, was the man behind the race, inspired back in 1980 during a training camp in New Zealand when he took part in the Round the Bays Race in Auckland where 20,000 runners took part.

There was nothing like it in Britain, though at the time plans were being hatched to stage the first London Marathon in 1981. Since then, the Great North Run has grown to become Britain's premier road race – although it was tinged with sadness for the 25th anniversary in 2005 when four runners died during the race. The coroner at the inquest which followed said there was nothing organisers could have done which would have prevented the tragedies.

Brendan, who will probably be better known for his association with the Great North Run rather than his achievements as an athlete which saw him win a 10,000 metre bronze medal at the 1976 Montreal Olympics, thinks the Newcastle race is so popular because "it fulfils people in a different way". He explained: "Society is getting soft and some people want to pull themselves out of that and say, I'll spend six months getting fit and I'll do that. Instead of watching from the sidelines, it's a chance to be where the action is. A few are trying to win it, some to finish it, some to raise money for charity, and some to run faster than they've run before."

For me the goal was a mixture of running well, getting a good time, and finishing without too much mishap. However, within a mile of the start, the call of nature fell my way. I couldn't resist it, and so in a tunnel, to the echoing

"Life is short... running makes it seem longer."

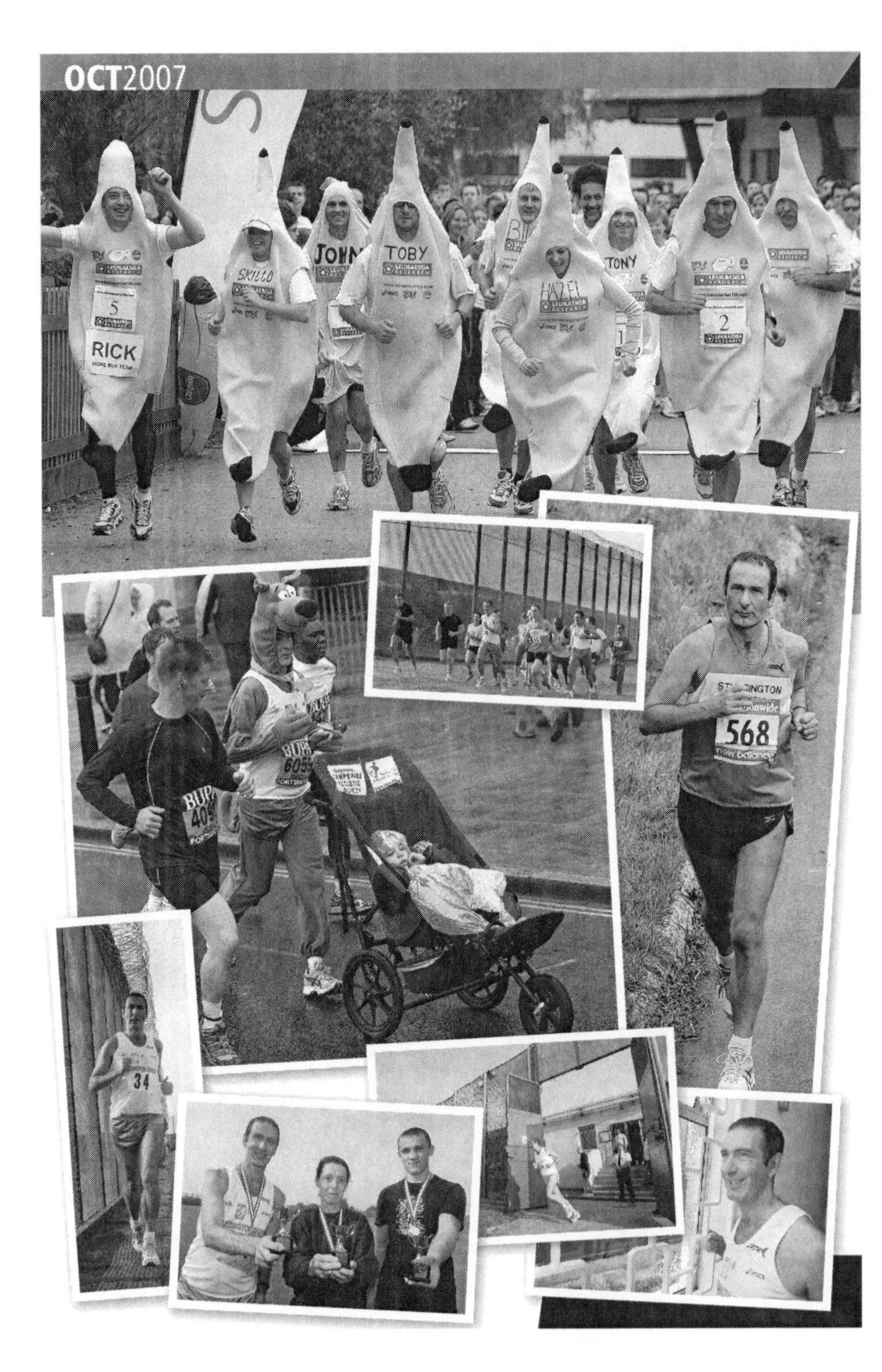
OCT2007
RICK
TOBY
JOHN
SKILLO
HAZEL
TONY
568
34

OCTOBER

62. Bananaman Chase 10k @ Milton Keynes

A NEW month and, to be frank, a total change of life. On October 1st I took up my new job as editor of the Swindon Advertiser; my first editorship and a heck of a challenge. That first week had passed me by like a whirlwind. It wasn't as if I could tread water and ease myself in to the job. No, the baton had been placed firmly in my hand and I was having to sprint hard.

The Adver was one of the few regional newspapers which had actually increased sales during the first half of 2007, so for the final quarter of the year I had the task of maintaining that year on year sales increase, as well as providing a fresh vision and motivation for my staff. It was a bit like a goalkeeper being brought on as substitute for the final 15 minutes to be told by his manager to keep a clean sheet! Besides, I was trying hard to remember everyone's names – not an easy task.

I was living away from the south coast having found lodgings in a house just outside Swindon, and then commuting back at the weekend to be with Liz and the boys. I missed them badly that first week so it didn't help that for the remainder of the year I would be working in Wiltshire during the week, and then seeing the boys briefly at the weekend before heading off for yet another race.

This first weekend of October took me to Milton Keynes – home of the infamous concrete cows which were made in 1978 as a leaving present from the Milton Keynes Development Corporation. These cows were designed by American artist Liz Leyh, who used recycled material and local school children to create them (the school children were used for assistance, not as materials). Since then these symbols of Milton Keynes have been stolen, had pyjamas painted on them, BSE graffiti scrawled about their bovine bodies and the cows even had to be rebuilt after they were beheaded!

My destination was Willen Lake on the outskirts of Milton Keynes for one of the more unusual races of the year. The Bananaman Chase was a major fund-raiser for Leukaemia Research. The idea of the 10km event was for competitors to chase 10 running bananas who had been given a five minute head start and see how many costumed characters they could catch around the two-lap circuit.

Earlier in the year, Leukaemia Research asked whether I would be one of those bananas tasked to run every kilometre at 4 minute 40 second pace, completing the distance in 47 minutes. How do you practise to run as a banana? Well, you're on the slippery slope straight away! I had never run dressed as a banana before so pacing was going to be interesting. The other nine runners were tasked to run at different paces – the first to finish in 45 minutes and the last in 1 hour 45 minutes.

There were a couple of old hands who had done this before and when it came to banana costumes they were ripe for advice. They told me to stuff some foam in the top of the outfit to prevent the head from flopping – I can't say I've ever experienced that running malaise before; floppy bananahead syndrome! Surely there must be a cream for that!!

The lead banana was TV actor and Emmerdale star Tony Audenshaw, who plays Bob Hope in the ITV soap. Tony is a lovely man. We had a good chat before the start about his work with Leukaemia Research and also his love of running. He has run a marathon in an awe-inspiring sub-three hours, and the previous weekend had completed the Great North Run in 1 hour 25 minutes. He is also the lead singer of a band called White Van Man and in Newcastle he performed at the Great North Run's running exhibition before running the 13.1 miles the next day. He's a very fit fella and an extremely nice guy to boot, who believes passionately about the Leukaemia cause.

Before the start of the race on a lovely October morning, Tony introduced each of the bananas to the 400 or so runners. I felt somewhat of an impostor to be there. Tony and the eight other bananas had close connections with leukaemia, their lives had become intrinsically woven with the disease having either lost friends or family, or battled through it themselves. There was John Reeve who raised over £100,000 for the charity by walking to the 2006 football World Cup in Germany in memory of his son Tim, who died of leukaemia in 2005, and there was Lindsey Skillington, who has raised around £210,000 for Leukaemia Research since her brother James died of leukaemia in 2002.

Leukaemia Research is the only charity in the UK dedicated exclusively to researching blood cancers and disorders including leukaemia, Hodgkin's and other lymphomas, and myeloma. Some 110,000 people, children and adults, live with these cancers today as 24,500 people are diagnosed with one of these conditions every year in Britain. The charity is committed to giving every one of them the best chance of survival thanks to scientists and doctors working at 50 research centres in the UK to improve the diagnosis of blood disorders and treatment for patients, as well as to find a cure for blood cancers. Leukaemia Research receives no Government grants and their life-saving research depends entirely on voluntary donations with the goal of raising more than £100 million over the next five years to sustain that investment.

The slowest banana was Hazel Staten who used to be a nurse and was diagnosed with leukaemia in Christmas 2003. She underwent chemotherapy, then had a bone marrow transplant with her brother acting as a donor. Since then, Hazel has been in remission, working tirelessly to raise money and awareness for Leukaemia Research. She is one determined lady.

Another person I met was four-year-old Jack. I was very nearly moved to tears when we met. "He should have started school last month but then things suddenly changed and we're doing our best to get by," explained his mum, who you could sense was beside herself with anxiety, but was trying not to show it to her young son.

Little Jack was diagnosed with leukaemia that summer and had already begun treatment for a disease which accounts for 1,200 children every year – about 80 per cent survive. Jack's hair was wispy thin and his eyebrows had disappeared – the result of intensive chemotherapy. A feeding tube had been inserted into his nose. "I'm going to catch you," said Jack, with a cheeky smile. "I bet you are," I replied, with a lump in my throat. When you have children of your own, the vulnerability of a young child hits home hard.

Jack and his mum joined the hundreds of other runners for the jog around the parkland course chasing myself and the fellow bananas. Of all the races I ran in 2007, this was the most humbling, this was the most sobering of experiences. I met others whose lives had been touched so dramatically and yet so tragically by a disease which seems to pick its victims at will. Their tales were heart-breaking, however it was also warming and uplifting to learn of their spirit and resolve. Some of the runners wore t-shirts carrying photographs and bearing messages for loved ones with the simple tag line: "in memory of…". I have attended a few of the Race for Life events organised by Cancer Research UK, the 5km women-only runs held during the summer which deliver a very powerful message about conquering cancer, as well as raising money to fight the disease. It's amazing how running can be such a powerful vehicle to draw people in this way.

At Milton Keynes, this was not a race where times mattered. It was about taking part. I had a blast, I really did. I showboated my way around the course, high-fiving with children stood along the route, sitting down on park benches to pose for photographs, telling Sunday morning walkers that no, they hadn't been drinking, they really were seeing a running banana, and I even managed to blag a carton of chips off a couple of teenagers sat at a park bench.

Every one of the 400 runners had fun around the picturesque parkland venue on a bright October morning, entering into the spirit of the occasion.

Despite being given a five minute head start, 16 runners managed to pass me as I stuck to the 47 minute goal. It wasn't easy running in a banana costume. Though the course wasn't too tough, bar one nasty little hill a kilometre after the start, it was warm and running was hard.

Trying to measure an even pace was also difficult; I was doing mental maths at each kilometre marker to ensure I was keeping pace. Incredibly, the first runner passed me after three kilometres - and I'd given the youngster a five minute lead to claw back. He eventually clocked 35 minutes for 10km.

I even had a sprint finish with one poor soul who must have been embarrassed to go head-to-head with a banana as everyone cheered us on to the finish, including a line of pom-pom-waving cheerleaders. The guy smiled at the finish, shook hands and told me how much it had meant to him to run for a cause which had also affected his family.

A great day and a great cause. A first for running as a banana with no slip-ups! I raced all over the country in 2007 competing in long distance runs and gruelling events, but this and the London Marathon were the only ones which moved me to tears.

63. IRC Haslar 10km run @ Gosport, Hampshire.

I HAVE never won a race before and I've never run inside a prison either! So here was two firsts in one day. The place was the ridiculously-named Immigration Removal Centre at Haslar in Gosport, Hampshire – surely only a small-minded, non-thinking Whitehall pen-pusher could have come up with such a crass name as the IRC.

Though it's not particularly something I like to brag about, I am no stranger to prisons. As part of my training to be a magistrate I have twice ventured inside the forbidding gates of Winchester Prison, and also the Feltham Young Offenders' Institute in Middlesex. These are two extremely depressing places, claustrophobic and where the sounds of keys being drawn and iron gates clanking shut echo throughout the building. The faces of the inmates are drawn, the eyes deep and hollow. I stood inside one cell chatting to a prisoner who was serving 10 years for armed robbery. He was sharing the cell which was about seven feet wide and 12 feet long, with another inmate. A corkboard by his bed held several photographs of his wife pictured with his cheeky-looking daughter. A couple of birthday cards were also pinned up along with some letters too. This was the depressing and sad human face of prison.

Once I also visited Kingston Prison in Portsmouth, a prison for lifers, where they have their own football team, the Kingston Arrows, which plays in the local league. They don't have any away games and if the ball is kicked over the wall no-one is able to collect it. I was invited to Kingston Prison a few years back to play in one of the inter-block games between prisoners watched by prison guards. Some of the players were inside for murder, so at first I was very careful not to make any late tackles. After a while you forgot you were playing on a football field inside this Victorian prison. The guys on both sides were good fun, and pretty good too. In fact there was less foul language and more sportsmanship on that pitch than I've ever found in a Sunday morning parks game.

But I digress. Having told friends and family that I won a race, and have a trophy to prove it, the cynics have come out of the woodwork. "Okay, how many runners were there?"

"Inside a prison? Surely the rest of the runners had a ball and chain around their ankles."

"Yeah, I bet the warders let you win." Envy, that's all it was!!

The occasion was a 10km race at the Haslar Immigration Removal Centre. It's not a prison as such, but as the title brutally suggests, it's a holding centre for those who have illegally sought sanctuary in the UK, waiting to either be deported, or resting on a decision whether they can stay in the country on the basis of political asylum.

Huge fences with barbed wire line the Haslar centre which is situated right on the Solent. CCTV cameras monitor every move, in fact to move anywhere within the grounds you had to pass through a series of gates.

However, that belies the fact that in the strictest sense Haslar is not a prison. The detainees are not kept in cells, but dormitories. Though they are not allowed out of the place, yet they enjoy a reasonably relaxed lifestyle with three meals a day, they have a gymnasium and education centre, and lights out is a pretty late affair.

The race was organised by the centre's gym department. This was the fifth year of an event which involves detainees, warders, their friends and family, plus runners from outside. Entry fees from the race go direct to charity. Fortunately for me, three of the fastest detainees had been released a week earlier. I'm surprised they weren't given the option to stay to take part in the race!

In fact only a few detainees took part in the race which involved little more than a dozen people, with several others taking part in a 10km walk. The race consisted of seven laps around the centre, starting on the sports field and wending its way along the perimeter walls, through gates and past the laundry, the kitchens and greenhouse, before finishing with a wide circuit of the sports field.

I am not a particularly fast runner, so with Mark Hindry, a fellow runner from Stubbington Green Runners, I wondered whether he would take on the pace, or if it would be one of the detainees. No-one did, so awkwardly I led from the start. Mark kept close on my tail, but I soon pulled away and was running quite comfortably on the circuits.

Other prisoners were there to cheer us on, along with warders. I passed a group of Asian guys who were ignoring the race, standing around chatting among themselves. I past them with the Islamic greeting As-Salāmu `Alaykum, (peace be upon you). Stunned by this they turned round to find out where the voice was coming from, spotted me and shouted back wa 'Alaykum As-Salām (and on you be peace). For the remaining laps they were my most enthusiastic supporters, waving and cheering me with "yala, yala" (go on, go on).

The sun was out and it felt strange to be leading a race. I wasn't bothered about winning, more of getting round without injury in this, my 63rd race of the series. I even pulled off the paths to take a longer route on the stone paths to ensure I didn't slip up on the wet and dew-ridden grass. With my new-found Arabic friends cheering me on, a couple even running alongside me for a few yards before giving up, the laps passed by and though the route was tedious – there are only so many laundry rooms and greenhouses you can pass - the atmosphere of the race was relaxed and fun.

Arms aloft, I crossed the finish line first in a time of 46 minutes 28 seconds, which must rank as the slowest winning time of any 10km race in the UK in 2007. Mark followed a minute later, and we applauded each of the runners as they came in.

Coming home in third place was Igor, a 24-year-old Ukranian from Novovolynsk, who found himself in Haslar waiting to learn whether he would be deported for holding a false passport. "I came to Britain on a student visa in 2005 working as a strawberry picker in Herefordshire," said Igor, who was arrested at a railway station with the passport which he picked up for £500.

"I was sent to prison, and now I'm applying for political asylum. I feel Britain is a much safer place. I fled the Ukraine because of all the guns and I fear for my safety if I go back home. Haslar is nice place to be. They are nice guys here although not everyone speaks good English."

Igor was fairly laid back and relaxed about his future, even though back home he had a 19-year-old sister, and both his parents were still alive. "I call home every two weeks, but I still want to make Britain my home."

He was delighted to have finished third in the race. "I still smoke, but I have been using the gym a lot at Haslar to improve my fitness," he added. "It was fun to have a race today, the longest I have ever run. Maybe I can get a bit faster."

64. Swindon Half Marathon @ Swindon, Wiltshire.

THE Swindon Half Marathon was never part of the schedule. In fact, the original plan was to run the Cabbage Patch 10 in Twickenham, a very popular race which is rated as one of the flattest and best 10-milers in the country. Back in 1993, Richard Nerurkar set a British record of 46 minutes 2 seconds for the race which is based at the Cabbage Patch pub, and takes in a route along the roads and towpaths through Twickenham, Kingston and Richmond.

I had already received my number for the Cabbage Patch 10, but then passed it on to a friend – a practice which is despised in some running circles, particularly the anally-retentive British Association of Road Races who, in one of their particularly dull newsletters that autumn, called for number-swappers like me to be banned because of the difficulties it causes to organisers for their results collation and potential difficulties in a medical emergency. "Despite years of trying to educate, persuade, cajole and frighten runners into towing the line, the practice of passing numbers on to other runners when the registered person is unable to run, still persists," they wrote in a newsletter which also featured a lovely double page spread of photographs showing how not to organise a race. Patronising and pedantic claptrap!

"Perhaps races should put a clause in their entry conditions stating that if a number is given to someone else (without the permission of the race organiser) and should that person suffer any illness or injury during the race, then the race organisers reserve the right to charge the medical costs to the runner and/or the original entrant," wrote Adrian Thiemicki, the permit secretary for Cheshire, who reckoned in one race that three per cent of the finishers weren't who they were meant to be.

Get a life guys! I found during the year that many races filled up very early – in one case, a Christmas 10km race was full by May! The drop-off rate is phenomenal. I don't have a problem with number-swapping so long as it is to a same sex runner, and that person puts their name and any medical details on the back of the number. Simple!

Fortunately, my mate Steve finished the Cabbage Patch 10 without an embarrassing heart attack, changing sex or causing mass confusion among the results compilers – though he didn't pay me back for the number, cheap skate!

However, with a new job in Wiltshire, it was hard to ignore the Nationwide Swindon Half Marathon, which is now in its fourth year and held on the same day as the Cabbage Patch 10. The Swindon Advertiser was one of the race sponsors so what better a way of finding out more about the patch where you are working – so long as it wasn't a Cabbage Patch.

Would this be just another fairly ordinary town half? Not at all. I was pleasantly surprised. The Swindon Half is brilliantly organised. There was loads of car parking to the south of the town by the huge Nationwide offices, and thanks to the council the whole route was closed off to traffic. It was a superb event. No cars, and their impatient drivers, trying to muscle their way past a gaggle of runners chucking out exhaust fumes.

The race started near the building society headquarters with a sharp uphill climb, but then headed out along the Marlborough Road and out into the country. The route was surprisingly hilly, heading up to Wanborough, through the lovely village of Liddington and then back into the town. There were climbs aplenty, but the route was sprinkled with scores of very enthusiastic spectators and loads of drinks stations.

The weather was good, and this was a wonderful race. I enjoyed myself. The runners alongside were chatty and friendly - which made a pleasant change. There were an estimated 2,000 runners taking part as I crossed the finish line in 1 hour 37 minutes, almost identical to my time at the Great North Run a fortnight earlier.

I was handed my medal by the leader of Swindon Borough Council, Rod Bluh. Exhausted, with a bit of dribble on my chin, and even a touch of bloody nipple rash appearing on my green running vest, I shook hands with Rod who I was meeting for the first time and said "Nice to meet you, I'm Dave King, the new editor of the Adver." This most important of people in Swindon, who I was to get to know better in the coming months, was left speechless. First impressions count, you know!

65. Bushy Park Time Trial @ Hampton Court, Middlesex.

A MIST hovered over the park as a stag, its antlers standing proud, foraged quietly amongst the trees. A cold snap filled the air as the sun tried to pierce a way through the low-lying mist. This could have been picture straight out of the desolate Scottish Highlands, but it was London, just a stone's throw from the River Thames.

This was Bushy Park, lying in the shadow of Hampton Court, shortly after eight o' clock on a chilly Saturday morning. Bushy Park is one the royal parks where deer graze. In fact, because of the recent foot and mouth outbreak, warnings had been posted around the park and disinfectant mats had been laid at the entrances.

Every Saturday morning, hundreds of runners gather for the Bushy Park Time Trial, a 5km sprint around the park. It started in 2004 with just 13 runners, that Saturday there were 336 for an event run totally by volunteers. This is a free event held every week where runners turn up and measure their improvement over a flat, off-road course, set in a beautiful environment.

There are similar time trials held around the country in Wimbledon Common, Basntead Woods, Rolf Valley, Richmond Park and Hyde Park in Leeds.

Before the race, I caught up with organiser Chris Wright who recalled how the idea had originated over a few drinks in a pub a few years ago with him and Paul Sinton-Hewitt. "The time trial has grown and grown," he said. "We wanted to organise something each week at the same time, a race over the same distance which would give runners a target.

"It's free, and with races today costing so much, maybe that is something which organisers of the so-called bigger races should think about."

Now top internationals such as Sonia O'Sullivan and Craig Mottram have also taken part in the Bushy Park event in the past couple of years mingling with club runners and joggers - abilities spread between those running 5km in 15 minutes to 40 minutes.

It has been a sensational formula and what a fantastic race. By the time the woolly hat and thermals came off come race time, the mercury on the thermometer was still hovering close to freezing and you could see your breath mix with the early morning mist.

There was a smattering of schoolboys from the nearby Tiffin School, runners from strong clubs such as Newham & Essex Beagles AC, Belgrave Harriers and Hercules Wimbledon AC, as well as a veritable feast of enthusiastic competitors.

The pace was quick and smart, and I was out of the blocks quickly; more than anything to keep warm. I was surprised and pleased with my pace. It was steady and despite not doing any speed training for the past year, I felt quick. I didn't look at the watch, but stuck with the pack on the huge loop around the park, trying to finish strongly picking off runners on the way in.

My time of 20 minutes 54 seconds was by no means my fastest 5km ever - but I was over the moon to be running that quick at this stage of the season with a succession of half marathons in my legs. The time was good enough for 69th place and afterwards it was off to trooping round the Hampton Court maze with my boys who had emerged from the car for the finish, lured by the attraction of a bacon buttie and a cup of hot chocolate from the mobile canteen which had positioned itself in the car park.

By this time, the mist had lifted, the sun was shining and the stag has disappeared. This was a stag do with a difference!

66. Stroud Half Marathon @ Stroud, Gloucestershire.

DRIVING to Gloucestershire on a cold and misty Sunday morning in October, the hazy view couldn't disguise the beauty of the Cotwolds.

Joined by Liz, we drove through delightful chocolate box villages, along twisting and turning roads dipping down steep valley roads before making a gradual climb out of these charming places.

And as we drove closer to our destination in Stroud for the town's half marathon I figured we were in for a tough 13-miler, littered with some devilish climbs and spectacular views. How wrong I was!

The Stroud Half is now in its 26th year, so is something of an established race. It's a heck of a walk from the parking spot by the railway station to Marling School, and once there the organisation was a little chaotic. There were huge queues for registration, longer queues for the toilets, and though the race was catering for an estimated field of about 2,000 runners, it had more of a school fair feel to it.

I just about managed to fight my way for a space in the small school changing rooms, strapped on the computer timing chip to my shoe, handed my gear to a lady manning the baggage tent and joined the rest of the throng on Cainscross Road for the start.

Word was that what lay ahead was far from hilly, so not to worry. And those predictions were proved right. The race headed out of Stroud towards Stonehouse and along pleasant country lanes past Standish Church before crossing the M5 just short of the six-mile mark.

Nothing wrong with the course, just plain and unspectacular, and it didn't get any better. We joined the main carriageway of the A38, turned back towards Stroud through Westend to the A419, took a loop through an industrial estate and then a three-mile run to the finish at the school.

It was an okay half marathon, but so uninspiring and, given the location, so disappointing. It would have been wonderful had the race been routed around more attractive parts of the Cotswolds and not industrial estates or busy dual carriageways.

A week earlier, Swindon, which I hadn't expected much of, had shown off its finest colours with a fantastic event which took in both the town and much of the beautiful Wiltshire countryside. One of the winners said afterwards that for some runners they would be put off by an event like Swindon because of the many tough climbs. "Too many runners enter races to chase personal bests, which is a shame," said the runner. Much could be said of the Stroud race.

It attracted a quality field up front, won by the Poole-based Zimbabwean Williard Chinhanhu in 1 hour and 6 minutes, but surely races are not about providing fast and comfortable courses.

Of course, there are safety issues and with police costs an important element, organisers are restricted about where they locate races, but surely it is more difficult to close off the lane of a busy dual carriageway than a back road in the rural Cotwolds.

I was happy with my run, nonetheless. I was running very consistently as this was my third consecutive half marathon run in 1 hour 37 minutes.

A few days later, I was at the Rose Bowl near Southampton, the home of Hampshire County Cricket Club, to host another of the fund-raisers for the Hampshire Autistic Society. Around 270 guests attended a celebrity Question of Sport evening which featured the Southampton Football Club legend, Matthew Le Tissier, Hampshire cricketers Shaun Udal and John Crawley, Davis Cup tennis star Chris Wilkinson and Olympic athlete Iwan Thomas. The event was sponsored by south coast recruitment specialists, Hudson Cooper.

The Saints' skipper, Claus Lundekvam, had been due to attend but half an hour before start time he was no where to seen. Matt called Claus on his mobile to discover the Norwegian defender was stuck back home in Scandinavia and unable to attend. So Matt put a call into Gordon Watson, another ex-Southampton footballer, who dropped what he was doing and at very short notice made up the sixth member of the team.

The evening went extremely well. First off was a quiz organised by a good friend of mine, Simon Tooley. That was followed by a question and answer session from the audience to the panel of guests which I hosted with radio presenter Peter Hood. There were some television cameras following Iwan around for one of those fly-on-the-wall documentaries, and the evening, besides being great fun, raised £6,000 for the Hampshire Autistic Society, as well as boosting the profile of the charity.

67. BUPA Great South Run

IT started as quite a good idea, but there was no accounting for the torrential rain or unremitting south-westerly winds which turned the BUPA Great South Run into one of the wettest and blustery ever.

The idea was to run in fancy dress at this showpiece event in Portsmouth to maximise publicity for the Hampshire Autistic Society, as well as to give myself something different to write about in my 80-race challenge.

Running as one of the David Bedford-like 118-118 characters had been an early thought – and there were a couple of those on the day - but then after seeing Hampshire cricketer Shaun Udal at a press call the previous month dressed as Scooby Doo, my mind was made up. What a great, eye-catching costume!

I managed to pick up a Scooby Doo outfit from a shop in Southampton, fashioning the garment to pull a running vest over the top as well as fitting running shorts - with a hole strategically cut through the shorts to allow the tail to peak out. I had also re-enforced the tail with coat-hanger wire to make it less floppy and more perkier!

The fashion attire was all a far cry from 12 months earlier when I had taken part in the Great South Run wearing normal running gear, only for the elastic to snap in my shorts half way round. The weather was also very wet that day, that horrible drizzle which sticks to your skin and permeates through your clothes no matter how waterproof they seem to be. This was a running first, a dilemma which no training manual will ever cover. What do you do when the elastic goes in your shorts in the middle race, and they start slipping over your hips?!!

Several friends suggested I should have just stripped off to my undies, running along the coast road to the finish at Southsea looking like an extra out of The Full Monty.

Instead I was forced into running repairs, snapping off a safety pin which was attached to my number, and linking together both my shorts and rain-sodden running vest. But this had very little effect. The safety pin gingerly held up one side of my apparel but the right-hand side of my shorts still slipped down. Meanwhile, my race number was performing kite-flying acrobatics off my vest as a sharp wind billowed off the Solent. I re-attached the safety pin back to the race number, resigned for the last few miles to running at a gentle pace, shoring up my shorts over my belly button every 30 seconds, once they had slipped down.

Twelve months on there were no such problems, not dressed in a Scooby suit, wearing just underpants to prevent any unnecessary chaffing. To make the 10-mile challenge even more interesting, the plan was to push my son Ross around the course in his specially adapted sports stroller. As the rain kept pouring while we sheltered in a car, I knew I couldn't opt out now. We headed for the start on Southsea Common ready and raring to go in the rain. I had to wrap up Ross in waterproofs to keep him dry as possible.

The Great South Run is a big party on the south coast, even in the rain. It is a brilliantly organised race – despite major problems which persisted on the railways that day – and though not as big as its Tyneside cousin, it is one race you don't want to miss for the carnival atmosphere along the route alone.

The sight of Scooby Doo pushing a sports stroller went down a treat. The response from fellow runners was great. They were full of encouragement. By the first mile I knew this was going to be hard. What I hadn't accounted for was Scooby's bouncing head which was out of control and kept flicking from side to side and into my face. Very soon Scooby's grinning face was whipping into my eyes and by the end this had left me with bloodshot eyes, as well as an awful headache.

Vision with the outfit was also considerably reduced, especially with pushing the stroller through the heavy crowds of runners. However, despite the decreased vision, my sore eyes and overheating in the costume in wet weather, this was more than compensated by the reaction I got around the course.

It was awesome. I felt 10 feet tall. For 90 minutes, wherever I ran there were cries of "Scooby Doo". Young children cried out, their parents would point and I'd wave back. Sections of the crowd would suddenly begin cheering as one when they spotted me. It was a fantastic feeling. Policemen on motorbikes, security guards in the dockyard, all offered generous words of encouragement as I pushed Ross along.

The raced route started on the seafront in Southsea, and then wound its way through Old Portsmouth and into the historic dockyard, past the museum where part of Henry VIII's ship the Mary Rose is housed, and beside both HMS Nelson and HMS Warrior. We looped through Portsmouth and then back into Southsea, before a final cut back from Eastney and along the seafront to the finish by South Parade Pier. I was going along at a fairly gentle nine minute mile pace and though I was starting to hurt with my eyes, I felt I was doing okay.

We passed one pub which seemed to be doing a brisk trade. The punters, glasses in hand, cheered us as Scooby and Ross hared past. I asked one lady whether I could share her drink, she answered back that the pub didn't serve dogs!

All was going well until mile eight as the course turned at Eastney and headed west back towards Southsea and the finish. As we rounded Eastney Barracks we were hit by a most horrendous headwind. Other runners described afterwards how bad conditions were, how it had been a battle for them over those final two miles.

For me it was even harder. Imagine running with your arms dropped by your side and just using your legs as power for an hour and a half. It was agony. With Ross's six stone getting heavier in the stroller as I became increasingly tired, I was struggling. I had no arm movement to power myself against the wind. The only power was from my legs.

It was hard and I had to grit my teeth. Where previously I had acknowledged the crowd's support, waved back, danced a jig to some of the bands along the route, even answering back some of the banter, for this final stretch I had no energy left. It was a tough battle.

The distance wound down...two miles, one mile, 800 metres and then 400 metres to go. It was the longest two miles ever. I seemed to be making hardly any progress at all, and I was continually being passed by other runners who sympathetically offered me support in the face of this brutal headwind.

Finally I entered the finishing straight the cheers from crowds gathered on both sides of the road by the Pyramids Centre were immense. I tried to sprint but I was spent. I crossed the finish line in 1 hour 34 minutes and I was exhausted. Marshals moved in to quickly put foil wrapping over Ross who seemed quite content and unmoved by the whole experience. Slowly and unsteadily, I moved through the finishing funnel so glad to have completed the Great South Run.

It was only 10 miles, but it was a hard 10 miles. It was wet, it was windy, and it was bloomin' tough.

"Running has never failed to give me great end results, and that's why I keep coming back for more!"

NOV2007

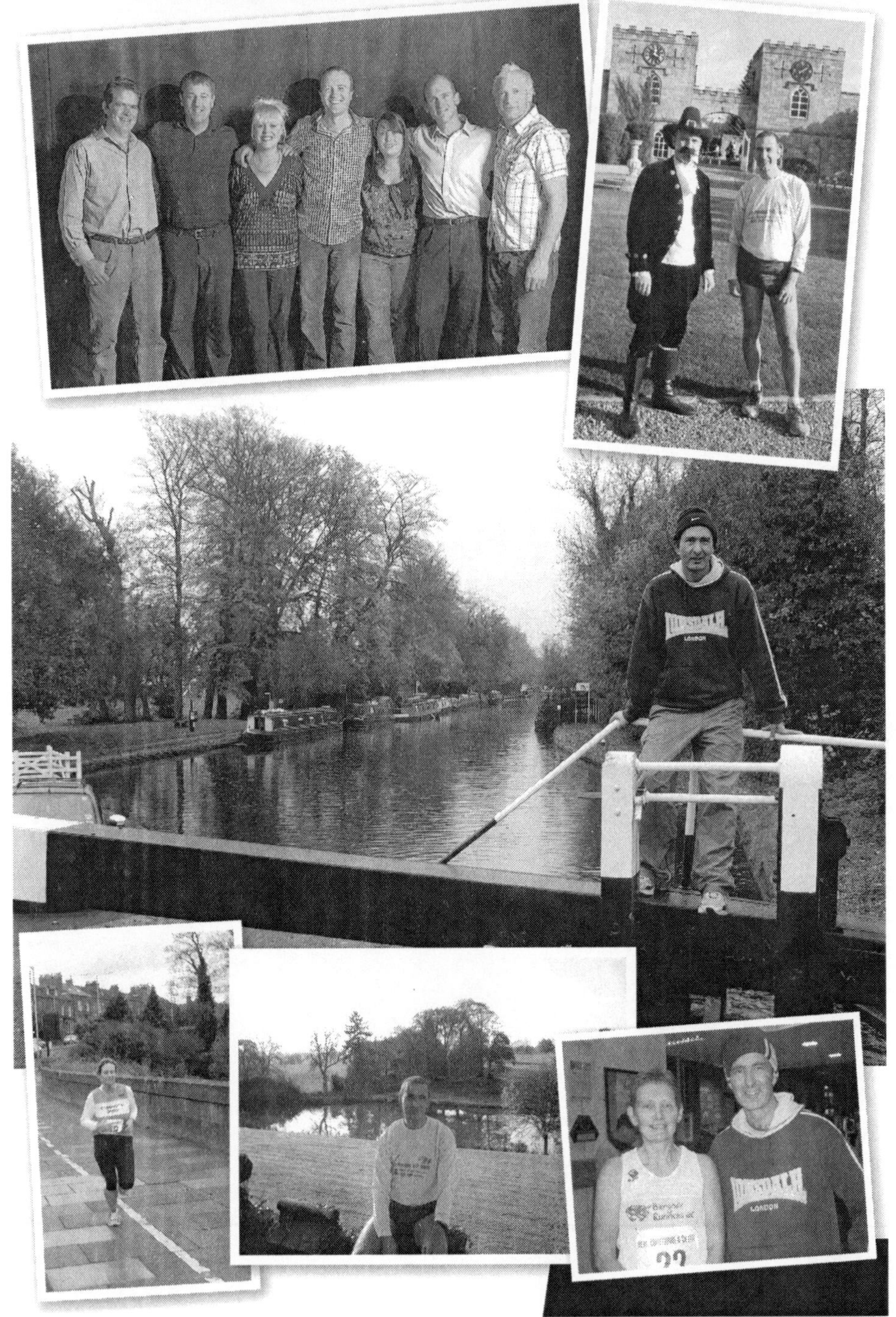

NOVEMBER

68. Guy Fawkes 10 @ Ripley, Harrogate, North Yorkshire.

WHEN it comes to Guy Fawkes and fireworks, Ripley Castle in North Yorkshire has got form. The picturesque pile, just north of Harrogate, has been in the Ingilby family for some 700 years.

According to the Ripley Castle website: "Our history is one of political, military, religious and social turbulence, of plague and persecution, of renaissance, enlightenment and industrial revolution. It is a tale of romance, courage, loyalty and recklessness. There is no final chapter because we are still here, still enjoying the adventure."

So what's the story? Well, Henry Ingilby collected taxes for Edward II helping the king to finance the construction of Windsor Castle, while his brother Thomas saved the monarch's life by killing the wild boar that was about to commit regicide. He was knighted for this noble act of courage. What a boar!

As for the rest of the family, Sir William Ingilby held high office serving Henry VIII, Mary Tudor and Elizabeth I through some of their darkest days.

Meanwhile, two of his sons toured the countryside inspiring rebellion and were described as "the most dangerous papists in the north of England". Francis Ingilby paid the ultimate price and was executed in 1586.

Most famously, "Trooper" Jane Ingilby whose portrait with the enhanced cleavage hangs at Ripley Castle, is said to have held Oliver Cromwell at gunpoint overnight in the castle when he had the temerity to advance on Ripley Castle.

But it is for the Gunpowder Plot that the castle has become synonymous, a daring plan which, if it had come off, would have killed the Royal Family and destroyed Parliament. James I actually stayed at Ripley Castle in 1603, but by 1605 the Ingilbys were plotting to kill him. In fact, nine of the 11 known conspirators of the Gunpower Plot were close relations or associates. Maybe the Ingilbys didn't like the fact that the King never helped with the washing up after the sumptuous feast, or perhaps he left the loo seat up on the royal privy!

So, what does all this historical nonsense have to do with running? Well, for the past 24 years Nidd Valley Runners has organised a Guy Fawkes 10 mile road race which starts outside Ripley Castle and finishes in the grounds.

It is a challenging run on quiet, country roads packed with plenty of no-nonsense climbs. A week earlier the weather had been appalling for the Great South Run in Portsmouth, but for the first weekend of November we had a crisp Sunday morning – a fresh snap, mingled with a clear blue sky and not a breath of wind – perfect running conditions.

Those fresh conditions gave me an ideal wake-up call after a 4.30am alarm call and then a 270-mile drive from the south coast to Yorkshire.

Originally, I had planned to head over to Kent that weekend to run the Deal 5. With all the long distance races I had been clocking up lately, this five-mile amble in Hop Country would have provided a spot of light relief, and ticked off one of the few counties which I had not visited so far. However, work commitments meant I had to be in Manchester on the Sunday evening, so not fancying a long haul up from Kent to Lancashire on a Sunday afternoon, it was a case of Deal and no Deal as I chose a race in the north.

The road through Ripley winds gently past a cobbled market square, an ancient church, market stores, old stone houses, village stocks and an old coaching inn. And in the centre lies Ripley Castle.

The bell from the church tolled as we set out on a beautiful November morning, sunny yet fresh, with not a breath of wind. A chap dressed as Guy Fawkes waved us off. I was very tired and lethargic for the start, a sluggishness which never passed.

The hills, four of them in all, were very tough. Two in particular offered steep gradients which reduced many to walking pace. I stuck grimly to the task determined not to stop, yet running within myself determined to enjoy the run while savouring the gorgeous countryside. It was a backdrop of splendid greenery as we ran along quiet country lanes, beside dry stone walls and fields with sheep, dropping off the hills into pretty Yorkshire villages. Classic Emmerdale country.

We swept up a woodland trail for the finish which turned into the grounds of the castle with a serene lake providing a marvellous backdrop. The goodie bag afterwards was a chocoholics' paradise. It was a lovely day for running and after the hard races of recent weeks it was nice to run without too much pressure enjoying the delightful countryside.

69. Grand Union Half Marathon

APART from the occasional muscle strain and odd niggle, I had gone ten months without injury. In fact, come early November I had run 615 miles and travelled 18,936 miles around the British Isles without even an ankle strain or an in-growing toenail. Credit was due to the fortnightly physiotherapy from my friend Mark Diment. The spitting image of comedian Lee Hurst, possessing a zany sense of humour to match, Mark is a guy with tremendously strong hands who, as soon as he sees your pelvis out of kilter, has it fully aligned several bone clicks later.

So after going out of my way for 11 months to avoid injury, what happens? I walked straight into a metal skip at work! Don't ask how it happened, this was an act of total muppetry and my only excuse was that it was dark as I walked into the sharp edge of the skip. I went to see the doctor who reckoned I had damaged two ribs close to the sternum. Ordinarily, rest should have been the order of the day to allow to ribs to heal. They hurt. Hurt big time. But there was no way I was going to rest right now.

Ideally, I would have preferred a gentle 10km race without too many hills at a nice even pace. However a half marathon was one race I didn't want facing me. Race 69 was the Grand Union Half Marathon from Cowley in Middlesex to Watford in Hertfordshire. This was 13 miles of running along a rugged, concrete towpath, sweeping under bridges, putting in short and sharp sprints up to lock gates, while dodging anyone coming the other way. Just perfect!

Friends had suggested giving the race a miss to allow the injury time to heal, but there was no way I was going to fall behind on my schedule with just 12 races and little more than seven weeks to go until the climax of this year-round running odyssey.

I dosed myself up with Voltarol, a pain-killer which always seemed to work, and which initially did the trick. But as the race wore on and my legs laboured, so my chest became painful. It was the breathing more than anything which hurt. The trick was to run slower, relax, breathing shallower without taking in huge lung-busting, chest-filling gulps of oxygen. The trick worked to begin with, but towards the end of the race as my body became fatigued so breathing was harder, and my chest felt as if it was cramping.

If the scenery had been more picturesque it would have taken my mind off my deteriorating physical state. But the Grand Union Half picked a dull and relentlessly uninspiring route.

The Grand Union Canal was once the busiest waterway in the country. It was the M1 of its time, a 137-mile route stretching from London through the Chiltern Hills, rural Northamptonshire and Warwickshire, and into the suburbs of Birmingham.

Today, the Grand Union Canal remains a busy, leisure waterway that has seen better times. A few of the barges were brightly painted, adorned with flowers, looking like floating Romany caravans. Yet some of the barges tethered to the bank had not seen a lick of paint for years. These rusting hulks are still home sweet home but a few were nothing more than grotty, dilapidated vessels lining the towpath. Floating heaps of rubbish.

The route of the race headed north through Uxbridge, under the A40 near Denham, past Harefield and onwards to Watford. For me, this was close to home. I grew up five miles away from the start in Ruislip, and it was on the Grand Union where I learnt to canoe – very badly.

From a running point of view, this was pretty turgid stuff. The towpath was dotted with unsmiling fisherman distinctly cheesed off that sweating runners were destroying their morning pursuit. We passed families out for a stroll, and owners dressed in grubby overalls carrying out repairs to their barges or tending small patches of garden. Occasionally wood smoke drifted skywards from the chimneys on the drab barges.

This was the first time the race had been staged. Most of the runners had initially gathered at the finish in Casiobury Park in Watford ready to be bussed to the start. When we arrived in Cowley, it was frustrating to find there were no toilets. We were told we could use the nearby garage or pub, which simply wasn't good enough. Not when we had paid £12 to enter and another £5 on top for the transport. It was fair enough for the guys who could find a quiet corner in the woodland for a constitutional, but for the ladies on a cold and drizzly start to the morning it could not have been comfortable.

The organisers, Purple Patch Running, one of the new breed of internet running clubs, weren't helped either when water from the first of three water stations at three miles was stolen!

The race finished back in Casiobury Park in Watford. I ran with an Irish lad for much of the way before he put in a sprint near the end. I was hurting so much with my chest that I couldn't respond. He was training for the Luton Marathon being held the following month, so straight after the 13-mile race he added on another eight miles by running home to Gerrards Cross. Nutter!

It was the first half marathon along the Grand Union Canal, and while this was an experience, it is one race in future which I won't touch again with a bargepole!

70. Brampton to Carlisle

AFTER 71 races I've collected my fair share of race mementoes. Besides the usual mugs, t-shirts and medals of all shapes, sizes and quality, over the past 11 months I have also picked up a sack of potatoes, bottles of beer, a beer mat, various bits of food and a lovely towel.

It's not cheap to enter the races either. The big races such as the Great South Run can cost £28 – and though some might decry that as too much to pay for a couple of hour's entertainment, the Portsmouth event is one which I wouldn't miss for atmosphere alone.

But ordinarily we're talking of anything up to a tenner to take part in races. And for that you expect a good race, sound organisation plus a decent memento. Why a memento at the end of the race? Well that's what is expected and is par for the course.

So it was to Cumbria for the latest stage of my exploration of the British Isles for the Brampton to Carlisle Road Race. The event, which is put on by Border Harriers & Athletic Club has form. It is the oldest 10-mile race in the country and in 2007 this was its 56th year. Throughout its history, some famous names have won here including Ron Hill, Jim Alder, Carl Thackeray and Steve Cram to help give the race a classic status. Back in 1989, Angie Pain set a British and Commonwealth 10-mile record.

It cost £8 to enter the race, a further £3 for the coach which took you from a sports centre in Carlisle to the start in Brampton, not forgetting another couple of quid for the car parking. Your bags were then bussed back to Carlisle from the school gym in Brampton where we changed ready for the race. But at the end of the event all you got from the organisers....nothing! Oh, a plastic cup of water, and you could fork out for a t-shirt, but as for a post-race souvenir; nowt, zilch, absolutement zero!

The poorest value race I have run in this year? You bet. It wasn't a great race either.

On one side of the route was Hadrian's Wall which we never saw. This stone and turf fortification was built by the Roman legions with stretches from Segedunum at Wallsend on the River Tyne to the shore of the Solway Firth – a total of 73.5 English miles or 80 Roman miles. On the other side of the race route was the River Eden which we crossed on the downhill run in to Carlisle. But the majority of the race was spent traipsing along the laborious A69 with traffic lumbering past.

There was just one drink's stop on route which bizarrely served warm water. That was a first and foul tasting it was too. Still suffering from the effects of my close encounter with the skip at work, I surprised myself by running 70 minutes for the distance despite being dosed up with painkillers.

That was the fastest I had run 10 miles for a year which was very pleasing, bearing in mind that training schedules had been sacrificed and I had not put myself through a speed session.

After the race, I bumped into Gay Eastoe who I spotted during the run because she had written a cursory warning on her running gear that she was an autistic runner. She had written a book herself about her experiences as someone suffering from autism – "Asperger Syndrome: My Puzzle". She lives in the Lake District with husband Richard where they have four children. "I was diagnosed in 2002 after experiencing severe panic attacks," recalled Gay. "An anaesthetic given for a hernia operation was the trigger which changed me back into the person I was as a child."

Gay, who has three university degrees, works as a volunteer at a special school for what she describes as "very special children". "I do what I can, which is mainly chatting with the children and helping when asked," she added. A member of Blengdale Running Club based in the Lake District village of Gosforth, Gay has run seven marathons and two 32-mile ultra races when we met that November.

For her, running was a release. It was an environment where she found her natural equilibrium She doesn't allow her autism to get her down, but faces it head on with physical challenges. She loves climbing mountains, and says she has conquered more than 600 of the 1,000 feet plus fells in the Lake District. She also loves swimming and has raised over £38,000 for her local hospice.

The race wasn't great, but the visit to the north-west was more than made up for by meeting Gay; an inspiring person who doesn't allow her autism to conquer her.

71. Gill Pimblott Memorial 5km Race @ Tyldesley, Manchester

WHAT'S funny about Johnny Vegas? Johnny, well known and loved for his shambolic and spontaneous stage persona, is not my cup of comic tea, his brand of taboo-breaking comedy stretches the boundaries just a little far.

So what do you say to a guy who you find yourself stuck in a lift with for 20 seconds. "Hey Johnny, why are you such a crap comedian? Have you ever thought of going on a diet and giving up drink?"

This was the Hilton Hotel in Deansgate, Manchester. I had driven straight back from Carlisle to Manchester and had managed to blag a couple of nights' stay at the plush hotel, much frequented by the city's glitterati.

Johnny, with a suit slung over his shoulder, was in town for a TV awards ceremony at the hotel that evening. A red carpet had been laid out at the hotel entrance where TV crews plied their trade interviewing an array of soap stars I didn't recognise. As I stepped into the lift, suddenly I was joined by the husky-voiced Michael Pennington aka Johnny Vegas. A nod of acknowledgement as he pressed the lift button for the executive floor was all that passed during our briefest of meetings. Heaven knows what he must have thought of me, shabbily dressed in a tracksuit and smelling like a fishmonger's having yet to take a shower from my race four hours earlier in Carlisle.

The Hilton Manchester Deansgate, occupies the lower 23 floors of the 47-storey Beetham Tower dubbed the "Canary Wharf of the north". Liz was with me for the trip as we were treated to a fantastic room offering a panoramic view of the city, and a luxurious room with mini bar prices to match! After a year spent traipsing round a range of B&Bs, it was wonderful to enjoy a little bit of luxury. Liz went shopping and later had a pampering session in the beauty salon, while I chilled out in a deep bubble bath. We then headed for dinner in the Podium restaurant and later to Cloud 23, the hotel's fantastic bar for a cocktail in the sky. This was the life!

Manchester surprised me. I guess I had viewed the city through cynical Coronation Street eyes – a typical southerner's jaundiced attitude. But there is little doubting that Manchester now rates as one of Britain's top cities, rivaling London in terms of shops, trendiness and sophistication.

The following day, it was back to business. I was in Manchester for a much more sedate race than the 10-miler in Carlisle, and yes, unlike the cheap as chips Cumbrian race, there was a medal at the end of it. This was the Gill Pimblott Memorial 5km race at Tyldesley, a half-hour drive just outside of Manchester.

The race was organised by Astley & Tyldesley Road Runners, which describes itself as "not just a running club, but a social club", and is held in memory of Gill Pimblott, a lady from Astley whose family are closely connected with the club. She died of cancer four years earlier. All the proceeds from the race went to Dr Harland's ABC fund at Wigan Infirmary which helps with the early detection of breast cancer.

This was an extremely low-key event held at Gin Pit Village with the Miners' Welfare Club acting as the headquarters. The village takes its name from the gin pit which existed close by. A gin pit was a shallow mine which had its winding wheel fixed horizontally. A horse, tethered to a shaft and walking round and round, was used to turn the wheel.

Tyldesley was a huge coal mining town and in 1850 there were about 12 mines within a mile or two of the town centre. By 1945, over 8,700 people worked at the Tyldesley coalmines, with more than 6,400 folk toiling underground. The town had its fair share of mining disasters. The worst was at Yew Tree Colliery in 1858 when 25 men and boys were killed by an explosion of a fire-damp. In 1939, five men were killed by an explosion at Astley Green.

Today the reminders of this once great industry can still be seen around Tyldesley such as the Miners Hall on Elliott Street, the Astley Green Colliery Museum, the Astley and Tyldesley Miners' Welfare Club, and the slag heaps which surround the town. Astley Green Colliery was the last coal mine to close in 1970. Gin Pit Village has now been taken over by housing developers.

We changed in the warmth of the miners' welfare club before stepping outside to the bracing cold of a chilly and overcast November morning. For liquid, I had a bottle of blackcurrant juice with me held in a small, see-through container which I carried round with me. Shortly before the race, I popped into the toilets where there was an old guy having a constitutional. As I turned round, I could see him trying to pour the contents of my drink onto his hands. "Excuse me, what are you doing?" I asked. "It's soap isn't it?" replied the man. "No blackcurrant juice!"

The 5km race consisted of one small and then one large loop over heath land beside the welfare club, running over land where once the coalmines stood. This was a gentle saunter along the muddy paths of Colliers Wood. It wasn't the most scenic of races, more a steady Sunday morning run-out, splashing through the puddles. The atmosphere was friendly and my trot round took 23 minutes and 3 seconds to finish the 5km without too much effort. Despite the toil of two races in two days, the rib injury was not too bad with the Voltarol kicking in nicely to only leave a slight discomfort. But the end is in sight with 71 races completed and just nine to go!

72. Leeds Abbey Dash

THERE was an audible depressing sigh among runners limbering up outside Leeds' Civic Hall when the annoyingly loud and sprightly female announcer revealed the model Nell McAndrew would not be starting the race. It was a shame since Nell was an ambassador for Help The Aged which was the main beneficiary of the proceeds from the Leeds Abbey Dash in her home city.

As I have mentioned previously in the book, Nell and I have got history dating back to her first-ever London Marathon in 2004 on a very wet and cold capital day when I was chased a fair way round the course by Nell and a couple of minders.. It was my mission not to be beaten by Lara Croft with the 32D bust, as the surge of crowd noise acted as a constant nudge that a man's dignity was at stake. Eventually, I beat Nell by less than three minutes, but just to prove her amazing achievement was no fluke, she went back to London 12 months' later and ran a 3 hour 10 minute marathon cool as you like!

So I had hoped that Nell would have been there on Sunday for the 10km race – only because I was hoping to grab a chat with her for the book – a race which has been running for 23 years and, with 6,000 runners taking part, was hoping to raise around £150,000 for Help The Aged.

It is a great city centre race which starts from just outside Leeds Town Hall on a fast course out of town to Kirkstall Abbey and back. Sadly, this year the race wasn't able to route through the grounds of the 12th century Cistercian abbey, so the course looped by the edge of one of Britain's best preserved abbeys, and a return to the city centre.

Some 6,000 runners took part in the race which also formed part of an inter-area match attracting some blindingly quick athletes from all over the UK. Shortly before the race, I bumped into an old friend Gerry North, who was managing the south of England squad.

The 1960s were a glorious heyday of British distance running. Ron Hill, Roger Bannister, Chris Chataway, Gordon Pirie and Bruce Tulloh reigned supreme on the cinder tracks, on the nation's roads, and across country. Britannia ruled the waves, well metaphorically speaking, or when the athletics tracks were waterlogged!

And what of Gerry North? Gerry who? Gerry was also a leading light during that golden era of the sport, but a lot less heralded. Track running was for the glory boys; Olympic Games, Empire Games, headline making showpieces. Gerry's preferred surface was on the road and cross country. He was a brave and bullish front runner, not afraid to take on his opponents.

Over cross country, he won national junior, senior and veteran titles. He was crowned senior champion in 1962, capturing the prestigious title close to the family home at the Agricultural Grounds in Blackpool.

Gerry recalled: "I outsprinted Bruce Tulloh. He had just come back from New Zealand where he had run a four-minute mile, and I beat him. It wasn't speed, it was strength at the finish. Bruce never forgave me for that. Every time we meet he always mentions it.

"Yes, I was an aggressive, confident front runner. I was unbeatable in road relays and would go at people from the start. It's not like today where everyone is too scared of each other. I held one of the stage records for the old London to Brighton relay which I'm proud of."

Gerry was twice crowned Inter Counties Cross Country Champion in 1960 and 1962. He represented Great Britain in road race events around the world, running six miles in around 28 minutes, has a 10,000 metre time of 29min 6sec, and once ran 48min 38sec for 10 miles on a black cinder track which gave him a world top 10 ranking in 1962.

Then Gerry was approaching his 70th birthday. He's still a fit-looking fella, though a painful knee injury had hampered his daily runs. A far cry from an era when he would train sometimes two or three times a day.

"You couldn't stop me," added Gerry. "We weren't bothered with diets and all these fancy heart monitors. I didn't do any stretching exercises, I just went out and ran somewhere in the region of 80 to 120 miles a week.

"I must have run nearly 700 races and I only had one injury, which was a hamstring pull which I did during a two-mile track race. But within two weeks I was racing again because my body was strong. I don't think runners are as strong nowadays. And remember this was in the days of leather spikes on the track which meant the inside lane on a cinder surface really got churned up, so by the end of a race you were running in lanes two and three!"

Gerry was surprised that with the advent of sports science that distance running in this country hasn't moved on. He talked about some of the great front runners like himself who got on with the job. Runners like Ron Hill, Brendan Foster, Nick Rose and David Bedford. "I always felt more comfortable at the front. I hated slow races. If a race was slow, I'd put the boot in. Like David Bedford, I didn't have a sprint finish, I'd make the running early on.

"I don't know why distance running is like it is, why the times today don't bear comparison with the times we were running. I think it is down to the coaches who are telling their runners to hang back and attack towards the end. I also think it is down to the runners themselves.

"It is a different world today. When we were youngsters, we ran or walked everywhere we went. I had one fella in my training group who kept turning up late to sessions. I asked him why, and he said because that's what time his bus left the end of his road. I asked him why he didn't run or walk to stadium, and he replied that all his mates would think he was stupid."

Gerry would have been impressed that the race was won in a time of 29 minutes. It wasn't the prettiest of runs, but from a personal point of view I didn't care, I was flying. I shouldn't have been but instead of taking one I took two Voltarol tablets along with the traditional pre-race banana and Lucozade drink, and I didn't feel a thing.

I couldn't believe how quick I was moving. I had not been able to train between races, so my fitness was based around around the runs themselves. I was through half way in 21 minutes, and felt comfortable pushing on the pace. The ribs felt okay. I kept my breathing comfortable, relaxing as much as possible while letting my legs do the running. Towards the end I tied up a little, but was delighted with the time of 42 minutes 34 seconds, which was just under two minutes outside my personal best.

The Leeds Abbey Dash is built for personal bests. An out and back course with an incline heading towards the Abbey, but which gives it back on the return. Now with a bit of training and speed in my legs, who knows how fast I can go?!

I was pleased with the run, delighted to have got another race under my belt. The only downside was going back to the car afterwards, having to wait 75 minutes for a repairman to come out from Blackburn to fix my car boot which wouldn't shut properly, held together by just a shoelace.

Just before the race in Leeds, I held my final major fund-raiser of the year which was a sportsman's dinner at the Hilton Hotel in Southampton. It was a fantastic event, compered by my dear friend, Will Feebery, a leading light within the Rugby Football Union, and featuring the then Southampton manager, and now Scotland boss, George Burley, Irish rugby international, Conor O'Shea and Hampshire cricketer, Shaun Udal.

It was a great combination. In between dinner courses, I conducted a question and answer session with the three guests and at the end the guests were able to quiz all three sporting legends. The evening provided a fascinating insight into their worlds of sport, and all three were charming characters with some fantastic stories to tell.

Shaun in particular was great, relating the story of how during a visit to the Udal home in North Hampshire, big-hearted England captain 'Freddie' Flintoff saw off his daughter's school playground bullies with a few timely words.

He also told the story of how his wife Emma decided to hide the shattering news of their son's diagnosis of autism while Shaun was on tour with England – only breaking the news on his return to England.

Shaun told the audience how son Jack, who was then three-years-old, had his good days and his bad days. "It's been a bit of an eye opener for us, but we're coming to terms with it," he said.

"He's still in the early days of being diagnosed as to where he is on the autistic spectrum. He goes to a 'needs nursery' twice a week and we get help one afternoon a week to try to progress him on his social skills. He doesn't communicate; he's still not saying anything. He still can't eat certain foods. It's a difficult time and it's tiring – my wife gets tired very quickly. It's hard work, but he's adorable and you've just got to be there for him. You just take every day as it comes.

"We're waiting to find out if he can be admitted into mainstream schooling, and hopefully things will become clearer over the next six to nine months. Some autistic children get to their late teenage years and then suddenly develop, but we just don't know. But something like 10 per cent of autistic kids never speak, and we're still waiting to find out what's going to happen with that. The most frustrating thing from Emma and my point of view is that we don't know what he wants sometimes; we don't know what's wrong with him. That's tough – and it's hard on Emma because she's there with him all the time."

"Running is one the best solutions to a clear mind."

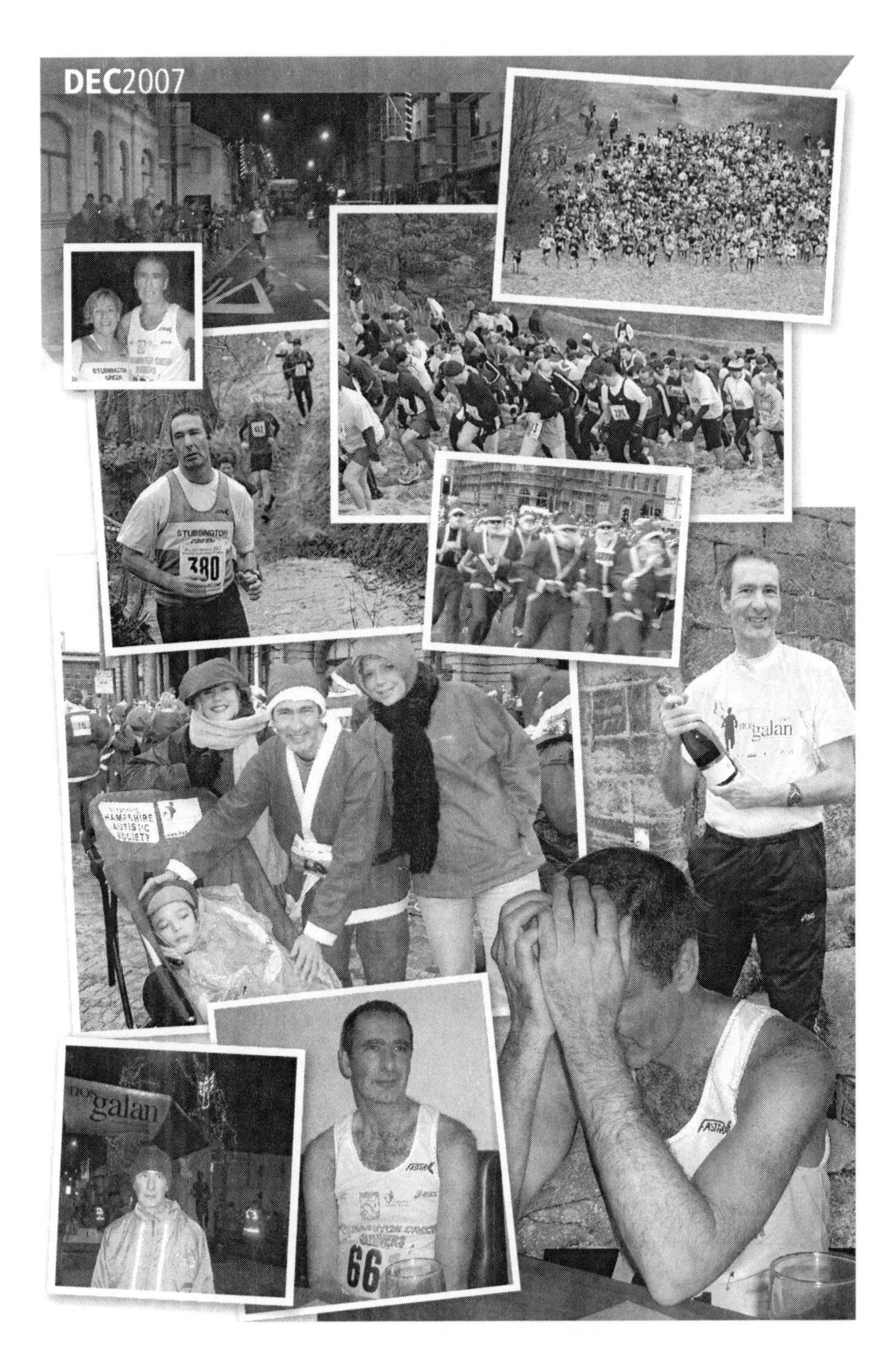
DEC2007
STUBBINGTON GREEN
380
HAMPSHIRE AUTISTIC SOCIETY
galan
galan
66

DECEMBER

73. Liverpool Santa Dash @ Albert Dock, Liverpool.

WITH more than 6,000 Santa Clauses milling about Liverpool on a wet Sunday morning in December, what a perfect time to commit a crime on Merseyside - dress up as Santa Claus, conceal your chosen weapon beneath the flowing red robes, use your Christmas present sack as the swag bag and replace unreliable reindeer with festive getaway car. Can you imagine the unfortunate victim trying to give police a description of the robber? "Well, he wearing this red hat, had a big white bushy beard, red outfit, and said 'give us your money, ho, ho, ho."

It was a truly surreal experience driving through the city centre where at every corner there were Santa Clauses of all shapes and sizes. Some were sheltering from the driving rain under the eaves of sodden buildings, others were standing on the steps of their hotel waiting for the weather to ease, while a few sat in Burger King to grab some pre-race nutrition. A minibus packed full of costumed Father Christmases passed us. We stopped at a pelican crossing, and a dozen Santas obediently sauntered across the road. One couple had a pair of dogs all dressed up with little reindeer antlers adorning their heads.

This was soggy Liverpool where 6,000 Santas ran through the streets of the city in a bid to set a new world record. The occasion was the Liverpool Santa Dash, held over a 5km course around the city centre which was aiming to raise more than £100,000 for charity.

Waking up in a Knowsley hotel early on Sunday morning, the weather was anything but festive. It was tipping it down outside, and a quick dash to the car in my cheap and cheerful Santa outfit discovered the weather was cold, and very wet.

I took part in the event with my son Ross in his specially-adapted sports stroller. He also had a Santa outfit to wear. I was concerned how much he might suffer in the wet and the cold while being pushed around. Also with us in Liverpool were Sally Hillyear and Gemma Harvey from the Hampshire Autistic Society, who had decided it would be fun to have a weekend away in Liverpool, to catch up on some Christmas shopping and to savour this Santa spectacular. What they hadn't counted on was the miserable early morning weather. Fortunately, by the time we arrived in the city centre, the rain had eased off and for most of the morning the streets remained dry.

It was classic comedy seeing so many fancy dress Santas. Anyone who had been out on the razzle the night before who had no idea what was happening in Liverpool first thing on Sunday morning must have believed they were still in a trance after necking a few too many sherberts!

We lined up for the race near the Albert Docks, and at 9.30am we set off on the 5km run. Progress was extremely slow. This wasn't a race, but a jog, and so Ross and I set off at a gentle trot. There was no point trying to get anywhere fast. We spotted Sally and Gemma taking photos by the start and pushed on. Many of the Santas were reduced to walking within a quarter of a mile of the start, and frustratingly chose to amble right in the centre of the narrow streets. So progress was difficult.

I soon got the hang of it as the route travelled around the side streets and thoroughfares of Liverpool. Ross and I soon picked up pace. We passed several people pushing youngsters in wheelchairs. We ran for a time with one fella pushing a disabled chap who was carrying a CD player blazing out The Pogues' and Kirsty MacColl's "Fairytale of New York". He was doing his best to get into the Christmas spirit.

There was a lovely, warm feeling to the race. Ross seemed content as for the final mile we were starting to pick our way through the field. We crossed the finish line back near the docks in 27-and-a-half minutes, the first pushchair across the line. The Hampshire Autistic Society got a mention over the public address as Ross and I finished, which pleased Sally and Gemma no end.

There was a t-shirt, medal and goodie bag for both Ross and me, before we headed off to Burger King, dressed in our Santa outfits, with Sally and Gemma to grab a hot chocolate.

For Sally and Gemma, it was interesting for them to see at first hand what it was like to live with someone with autism. Both are dedicated to the charity spending a lot of time working with those with the disability and their carers, but for Gemma especially, who had been with the organisation for less than a year, this was the first time she had spent 24 hours with an autistic child. We travelled up to Liverpool together on the Saturday morning, and headed for the Adelphi Hotel to collect our Santa costumes before Sally and Gemma embarked on some shopping. Gemma, who was so cold and desperately needed to buy some gloves even joined the huge queues outside Matalan. "I've never queued for Matalan in my life before," she said.

Ross was wonderful. He has a gluten and casein-free diet which his mum and I introduced five or six years ago. Gluten is a protein contained in foods such as wheat, barley, rye and oats. Casein is also a protein and found in dairy products such as milk, ice cream, cheese and yogurt. No-one quite knows why a gluten and casein-free diet helps so many autistic individuals, though thousands do so. Here's the technical bit, but in the intestinal tract, gluten and casein breakdown into peptides and these peptides then breakdown into amino acids. The peptides act like morphine in the body which can also pass through the blood-brain barrier and have a negative impact on brain development.

When Ross was four, I attended a talk given by Paul Shattock from the Autistic Research Unit, at the University of Sunderland, who has carried out a lot of research into the science of the diet. He remarked how a few days after removing gluten and casein products from an autistic person there seemed to be a period of regression – feelings of anxiety, clinginess, and over-affectionate behaviours, crying, dizziness, increased urination, even aching. But with the diet there was an improvement in the condition of children who had better concentration, better sleep patterns, reduced aggression, improved communication and co-ordination.

Basically, the diet works for Ross. What I and Ross's mum know is that the diet has had a positive impact on our son. He's far more lucid, his eye contact is good and his interaction impressive. Take away the diet, and Ross creeps into his shell. He regresses considerably.

As a result, it means he has a very precise diet, sometimes bland. Never mind the nappies, the videos and books, and a suitcase of spare clothes, but from a diet point of view going away, such as with trips to Liverpool, is a major logistical exercise. I had forgotten, for example, Ross's dairy-free yoghurts so trying to find them in a local store was very difficult. I had brought some pre-prepared meals with me to Merseyside which could be heated up for him.

On the journey north, Ross had his Thomas the Tank Engine DVD playing, and Gemma kept him occupied with his Thomas and Mr Men books. He can't talk, he can't read, but bizarrely every time Ross picks up a book he holds it the right way up, and will flick the pages from left to right. He does it every time, so clearly he recognises the words and shapes. I often wonder what lies inside his head, what is waiting there to be released.

Ross's quality of life is good. Later on in December, Ross's school held a Christmas service. St Francis School in Fareham, Hampshire, looks after children with a range of severe disabilities. When I visit Ross in school I see some of the other children who do not enjoy a great quality of life, despite the tremendous love and care from their families. Sadly, every Christmas, the head teacher lights a candle during the service for those children who passed away during the previous year. It is a very sad and touching moment. Though I sometimes feel a sense of frustration at Ross's autism, that his potential is not being fulfilled, I thank God he enjoys a good quality of life, he can laugh, he can run and he can show love. I could ask for no more.

As for Gemma and Sally, they said afterwards how they had learned a lot from spending time with Ross and they had enjoyed the time too. Ross is very responsive, not a typical autistic trait, but a rewarding one all the same. He is a beautiful and wonderful little boy.

Sadly, Liverpool's attempts to set a world record for the biggest gathering of Santas was beaten a few days later by Las Vegas which held a similar race attracting 7,123 festive runners.

74. Keyworth Turkey Trot @ Keyworth, Nottingham

WITH the finishing line in sight to my 80-race challenge, so the tension grew. After Keyworth, it was 74 races down, with six to go. Now there was no way I wasn't going to complete this epic journey. I had told friends that even if I picked up a major injury in the final few weeks I would take pain-killing injections to limp over the line if need-be.

But standing on the start line in Nottinghamshire, there was no hiding the pressure. It had not been the greatest week for me from a personal point of view, with plenty of distractions and worries. Earlier this month, my wife gave me the wonderful pre-Christmas news that she wanted a divorce. Her timing, as usual, was impeccable. When you're running you can't but help carry those worries with you. The divorce and the impact of it hit hard. For me, I had given a commitment, and though we had been separated for some three-and-a-half years, I felt that divorce was a sign of failure. I felt very bitter and depressed. These kind of anxieties loom large when you're struggling in a race, when the seeds of doubt appear, when your body is feeling lethargic and questioning whether you want to go on. You can't hide them. You ask yourself why am I doing this? Surely there are better ways of spending a Sunday morning than traipsing round a wet country lane.

Keyworth is a little village just outside of Nottingham and I was in the East Midlands for the Turkey Trot Half Marathon. This was the final 13-mile run of the year. After this for the remaining six races there was nothing more than a couple of 10km races. Get over the Turkey Trot and it really was plain sailing to the finale in Derbyshire on New Year's Eve.

After seven miles on a blustery Sunday morning in the East Midlands, I was running ragged and going through the motions. The course was hilly and challenging, yet it was the type of terrain I enjoy. But I couldn't get going, my mind was elsewhere weighted down by the anxieties, and I couldn't wait to get this race out of the way.

Then, out of the blue, our small pack of runners was passed by a disabled runner wearing a pair of carbon fibre transtibial artificial limbs - similar to those worn by Blade Runner Oscar Pistorius. Oscar was born with fibulae in both legs due to a congenital condition. When he was 11 months old, his legs had to be amputated halfway between his knees and ankles. The South African is fast, very fast, and at the time of writing he was hoping to compete in the 2008 Beijing Olympics using the J-shaped carbon-fibre prosthetics called Cheetahs.

There has been much criticism that the upside-down question marks give the 21-year-old sprinter an unfair advantage, since the blades are longer than necessary, allowing Oscar to cover more ground with each stride. The other important point is that Oscar doesn't suffer with the same lactic acid build-up which slows down ordinary athletes.

Whatever your view, it was amazing to see these prosthetics in full, flowing motion. The chap scorching past us in Nottinghamshire wasn't Oscar, but he was going at a fair lick. I was running with a small group of runners at the time. As Blade Runner passed we looked at each other in wonder at this amazing runner. "Well, at least he doesn't have to stop to tie up his shoelaces," was all I could say.

We weren't running slowly. However, this chap eased past, the blades just skimmed across the Tarmac road. I felt as if I had been left standing, and that moment gave me the massive kick up the backside I needed. I don't know who he was. He was too quick and was off and away before I could engage him in any post-race conversation. The organisers weren't too sure either as to the runner's identity, since he had entered on the morning of the Turkey Trot.

"Unbelievable!" said one of the runners in the pack. "The guy's got guts. How does he run so quickly?" said another.

Seeing Blade Runner soar past was uplifting on a tough hilly course shrouded by leaden skies and a cold wind whipping off the South Nottinghamshire Wolds.

The route of the Turkey Trot, which was celebrating its 25th year, took us mainly down country lanes and through picturesque villages. As I began to enjoy the race, I picked up the pace and the miles were very quickly rattled off.

There has been plenty of controversy in the sometimes anoraky world of running about the use of iPods in races. So many more runners are now competing with mobile discos blasting in their ears. For many they are a blasted nuisance and have been banned by some race organisers. In Nottingham there were many in evidence.

I had to give one iPod-wearer a nudge when she blissfully ran into me along a narrow country lane. Others were weaving across the road, ignorant of those around them, unaware of cars behind them or able to hear the marshals' instructions.

It was music to my ears when we finally headed back into Keyworth, passing the 12-mile mark on a downhill stretch into the village.

For the leading finishers, they each received a prize turkey. I finished 195th from a field of 762 runners in a time of 1hour 38 minutes 6 seconds. I felt like a prize turkey, but was glad to have wrapped up race 74. The end really was in sight.

75. Merthyr Mawr Christmas Pud 10km

STANDING at the foot of the Big Dipper – an enormous sand dune with a monstrous 245-metre climb – the first thought which seeps into the mind is "Oh, sugar!" ...or something like that.

The Big Dipper is Europe's biggest sand dune and can be found in Merthyr Mawr, just the other side of Bridgend.

Merthyr Mawr is an idyllic little settlement, as picturesque as they come, with an outstanding collection of thatched dwellings straight from the pages of a Thomas Hardy novel. With a wonderful backdrop of meadows and woodlands, the ancient Church dates back to the middle of the 19th century.

But Merthyr Mawr also packs a big surprise. It is surrounded by a huge network of sand dunes which stretch along the coast towards Porthcawl and the Mumbles.

It was here that the 1962 movie epic Lawrence of Arabia was filmed, although the weather on race day in December 2007 was more Siberia than Sahara. A biting wind blew off the coastline a few miles distant.

More notably, it was also in Merthyr that the likes of the great middle-distance runners, Steve Ovett and Steve Cram, would train, slogging their guts out on the soft and unremitting sand of South Wales. A few days earlier, I had met Christine Benning, an Olympic runner who competed for Great Britain around the same time as Ovett. "Merthyr Mawr? You're kidding," she said. "That is going to be hard work, believe me!" Geez, thanks for the pep talk!

Arriving at Merthyr Mawr I walked straight to the start where I saw the Big Dipper and could see exactly what Christine meant. This wall of soft sand just stretched skyward. If it had been Tarmac it would have been a tough climb. Around me, several runners arrived in festive fancy dress and set out to make the climb without a Sherpa or packed mule for a pre-race recce. "Whoa, that is one bitch of a climb," said one guy dressed in a Santa outfit. "That is gonna hurt."

Around 700 runners turned out for the race, many dressed festively for a party on the sand. Me? I wasn't in a mood to muck around with costumes, I wanted to blitz this bastard and get it out of the way. The running itself was no fiesta but the atmosphere was lively and fun, with fancy-dressed marshals also getting into the pre-Christmas spirit. At the one and only drinks station positioned after three-and-a-half miles, we were offered a choice of water or mulled wine and a mince pie. Now that was a first! Shame there was no brandy cream for the mince pie!!

But back to the Big Dipper and what a beast! It's part of a network of dunes which rolls towards the coastline at Porthcawl. The name Merthyr Mawr means "great tombs" referring to the large Stone Age burial complexes which lie beneath the million tonnes of sand.

The climb itself takes a good three minutes. By the time you reach the summit your lungs are burning as you are reduced to a walking pace. The soft sand saps every ounce of energy from your legs. With the massed start at the foot of the Big Dipper there was a sea of arms and legs as sand was kicked up everywhere. For those who get a clean start at the front on fresh sand, the climb is a little easier. Not so when you are sandwiched sardine-like between a mass of bodies scrambling ungainly up the slope trying to get a foothold and resisting the temptation to fall backwards. The sand churned up and was flying everywhere. It was difficult to get a grip. This was a knee-jarring slog.

The view from the top was fantastic, one from where you could just about pick out the coastline. Here there was something of a bottleneck as, for the next few minutes, the surge of runners squeezed down a narrow path which took us along the ridge of the dunes. My first mile took a snail-like 13 minutes before we eventually freewheeled down the other side of the dune. I wish I had bought a toboggan! Careering down the soft, bouncy sand was a piece of cake. This was fun, and the race suddenly became fully deserving of its title as one of the best 10km races in the country according to polls in the Runner's World magazine.

You're not going to run fast, not with the Big Dipper, plus a couple more tough climbs which greet you. However the delightful scenery and rural setting was fantastic. We ran down a quiet country lane as the bell from the nearby St Teilo's Church tolled mournfully. The course twisted and turned, crossed the Swing Bridge, curved round the back of a golf course, took a gentle downhill and then headed back along the estuary of the River Ogmore, which flows through Merthyr Mawr. The only penance was being tasked to run through two ankle-high icy streams with the finish line in sight.

Though the race labels itself as a 10km – 6.2 miles in old money – the true distance was a little bit shorter according to my Garmin watch. Hot soup and fresh rolls awaited every finisher, plus a bountiful goody bag including a Christmas pud. What a race, what hospitality – what a sand dune!

76. Christmas Pudding Dash @ Battle, East Sussex.

THREE days before Christmas, and the end really was in sight! It's funny how, during the summer, I couldn't wait to hear the first of those insanely annoying Christmas TV adverts, or to witness Christmas cards and decorations appearing in the shops. To me they were like the first drops of snow. Christmas is coming, and with that the end of this amazing journey around the British Isles.

Fortunately, I had already done my Christmas shopping, wrapped up all my presents and could skate off to East Sussex guilt-free for a Saturday morning jaunt

The place was Battle in East Sussex, some five miles from Hastings and the site where William, the Duke of Normandy, defeated King Harold II in 1066 at the Battle of Hastings. Now the town is centred around the Abbey, founded to commemorate this historic event which saw the Frenchman crowned William I, and which was dedicated in 1095.

But that's not all the history. A few miles outside of Battle lies Ashburnham Place. Set in idyllic grounds extending over 220 acres, it is now used as a Christian conference and prayer centre.

The grounds were designed and constructed in the mid-18th century by Lancelot 'Capability' Brown who laid out the three large lakes which encircle the house. He also built the Orangery, which is home to a number of interesting and unusual plants, as well as the oldest camellias in the country

The whole area looked spectacular on a frosty December morning with the lake frozen over and an ethereal mist hanging in the air. It was spectacular.

The area is rich in wildlife and part of it has been designated as a Site of Special Scientific Interest because of the valuable flora and fauna. That didn't stop organisers from hosting a five-mile multi-terrain race around the stately home grounds.

More than 200 runners and joggers lined up on a crisp Saturday morning for the two-lap race. There was a children's race beforehand. Gathered on the gravel path outside the stately home, we enthusiastically applauded all the young finishers and their chaperoning parents, before setting out ourselves on a tough, little course, with a nasty long hill midway through each of the two laps.

I started off at a suicide pace with a 6 minute 26 second first mile. A friend of mine, Paul Hammond, a team-mate at Stubbington Green Runners, caught me up by the first mile as we stepped off the tarmac and into woodland where it was muddy and treacherous. Paul, in fact, chose to walk up the tricky uphill stretches, but then zoomed past me on the flatter sections.

It soon warmed up and I felt a little overdressed with a thermal top and a running vest on top. The race had a lovely downhill stretch towards the main house at Ashburnham Place, and then it was onto the second lap.

Paul and I played a bit of ying-ing and yang-ing on the uphill stretches, but he finished a good half a minute ahead of me at the end. A wonderful setting for a Christmas fun, a lovely atmosphere, and a nice, gentle run-out.

77. Round the Lakes 10km @ Poole, Dorset.

AT £5 million a pop for real estate, Sandbanks in Poole has been described as a millionaire's playground – an oasis of affluence on the Dorset coastline with stunning views across to The Needles.

I'm not sure if Portsmouth Football Club manager Harry Redknapp was at home on Boxing Day morning with his Pompey team preparing for their evening clash with Arsenal.

Had he and wife Sandra gone for a brisk early morning constitutional, they may well have caught sight of hundreds of runners in their neighbourhood taking part in what has become one of the most popular 10km races on the south coast at this time of year.

The Round The Lakes 10km doesn't actually veer too close to Sandbanks to put locals off their festive Bucks Fizz breakfasts, but instead the race plots a four-lap route around Poole Park and the boating lake, with a final loop around the cricket field.

Such is its popularity that the race full signs were posted a good hour before start time with several runners, who were hoping to blow away the Christmas cobwebs by entering on the day, facing a frustrating and fruitless journey.

I again took the opportunity to run round with my son Ross in his pushchair, which wasn't too easy along some sections. We started off steadily and made good progress from the back of the field through the runners.

It was hard going at times, negotiating the speed bumps, coping with some impatient drivers in their gas-guzzling cars trying to edge past the runners, and pushing up one long hill which got harder with each assault.

Ross seemed to enjoy himself. Thankfully there was no rain and conditions were warm. It got a bit hairy by the end of the second lap when we were lapped by the front runners, some of whom arrogantly pushed past demanding other runners give way. There are ways of asking, and ways of asking.

We've all heard about road rage, but running rage? C'mon! This wasn't quite running rage, but a few years ago I ran a 10-miler along tight country lanes around Hayling Island in Hampshire. I was in a pack of runners including this mad woman dressed all in black. We were going at a fair lick so any abrupt changes of pace or direction was potentially hazardous.

Anyway, the woman in black was running all over the place like a drunk who had been turfed out after closing time. If I didn't know any better it was deliberately targeted as she cut me up on bends, and was running so close I'm sure she could smell the Old Spice aftershave.

Then she dropped behind me only to clip my heels causing me to stumble, and said nothing. Moments later, the same thing happened, but this time I was like Chelsea's Didier Drogba taking a swallow dive in the penalty area. Woman in Black had decided to run around me, and in doing so had taken the legs from under me. I tried to stay up, but crashed to the floor. I wasn't injured, bar a small graze on the knee. I was more angry than anything. The woman looked behind and said "Are you alright?" That was it - I just gave this woman a right mouthful. She said nothing. A complete nutter.

Anyway, back to the Poole race, and once the speedies had passed, Ross and I settled in for the final stages. The course got a bit repetitive towards the end. I was losing count of the number of laps we had run, but we crossed the finish line in a respectable time to grab our festive bottle of bubbly.

Seventy-seven races down, just three to go – I could smell the finish line.

78. Maldon Mud Race @ Maldon, Essex.

PICTURE this: it's a cold Sunday morning and you're on your hands and knees crawling on all fours across the mud flats of a river estuary. The rotting vegetable smell is retching, the feel of the gloopy mud presented in various shades of brown makes your skin crawl and you require the ability to control your nerves with the mud clinging to your body, trying to suck you under.

This was the Maldon Mud Race, a barmy escapade across the River Blackwater in Essex. I joined 180 other souls for what amounted to a crawl from Promenade Park, across the river along a route marked by flags to the saltings, then a short slog running parallel to the Promenade before a final exhausting shuttle back across the river bed to the finish.

Of course, the race took place at low tide although there was still a 30 metre stretch of waist-high water to be crossed. Fortunately, marshals in wet suits from the Chelmsford Sub Aqua Group were on hand to help any potential drowning victims.

In total, the race distance was around 450 metres and watched by several thousand spectators crammed on the promenade wall it was a gruelling slog.

The race began in 1973 following a dare waged with the landlord of the Queen's Head pub in Maldon. The challenge to the landlord was that the regular wanted to enjoy a meal served on the River Blackwater saltings while dressed in a dinner jacket. The challenge was accepted and completed.

The following year, a bar opened on the saltings when 20 locals made a mad dash across the River Blackwater, drank a pint of beer and slogged their back to the shore.

This was the start of the Maldon Mud Race, although in the following years so many people wanted to take part that there was a logjam on the saltings with people drinking their pint of beer.

So the alcoholic side of the race was scrapped and the mud race became a straightforward dash across and back.

The race continued from the Queen's Head until 1989 when the Maldon Mud Race ceased, but because of public demand it was revived in 1994 as part of the Maldon Carnival Association's calendar of events and run in conjunction with the Lions Club of Maldon.

So on Boxing Day, 1994, 52 people took part in the race which started and finished from its new venue in Promenade Park, with around 5,000 people watching from the shoreline. This event also raised more than £2,500 for local charities.

The race suffered a temporary blip between 1998 and 2000 when the Maldon Carnival Committee decided to abandon the event because of safety concerns. However it has now been run throughout the new century by the Rotary Club of Maldon and the Lions Club, and in recent years more than £100,000 has been raised for good causes in Essex.

For the 2007 staging of the race, it attracted a host of weird and wonderful costumes - several Santas, fairies, there was Spiderman, kilt-wearing Scots with ginger wigs, someone dressed up as a horse and his partner wearing a rider's outfit, a fella in a dinner jacket, some blokes wearing these inflatable Sumo outfits, and one lady even carried round a palm tree. Mad, absolutely barking!

I chose to dress in the top and bottoms from the Santa outfit which I wore in Liverpool earlier this month. It was disposable. Also, for the first time in this running challenge I wore football boots which were heavily taped up to my ankles to prevent them from being sucked under by the mud.

Just before the start, one guy who is an old hand at the race gave me the best possible advice: save your energy and don't try to walk through the mud, it will sap your strength - just crawl, he said.

A mud-fight between competitors shortly before the off got everyone dirty and in the mood, and then it was the start. We waddled down to the river bed and across the icy cold water. The first task was to climb up the sloping river bed on the other side of the channel. It was so hard to get any momentum going. Everyone was scrambling, clinging onto each other for support, pushing each other up the slope.

Walking was futile. You had to get on all fours and crawl. The mud crept to the top of your arms, you had to lift your head out of the way for fear of getting a mouthful. The smell was awful, the mud was bitterly cold too. It was hard, it was exhausting, and it was slow progress.

I managed to get to the saltings, and found a solid piece of ground on which I could walk slowly, before plunging myself into the mud for the return crossing.

It wasn't frightening, yet I wasn't comfortable stuck in the mud. My clothes were being weighted down my trouser bottoms were slipping off and I had to pull them up to keep them on. We clambered down the slope into the water, managed to walk across the river bed, and with the huge crowds cheering us on, plus a battery of newspaper and TV cameras filming our progress, we pushed on for a final surge/crawl to the finish.

Sad as it was, but my mud-splattered watch recorded a time of 10 minutes 17 seconds for the distance. The winner was home a good couple of minutes ahead, while some of the other competitors would take another half hour to finish.

There were cold showers waiting for us outside the finish area. I stripped off to shorts and a t-shirt, throwing my Santa outfit, football boots and socks in a bin. I managed to grab a second hot shower in the public changing rooms. The mud was clingy and horrible, as a sea of brown dirt ran across the changing room floor. Pity the poor person who had to clear up afterwards.

I walked out of the changing room and back to the car smelling like a skunk, my fingernails crusted with mud and my skin still covered with a film of grime. "Don't worry about it mate," said one fella. "It will take at least a couple of days for the smell to go! You'll be smelling the River Blackwater on New Year's Day!!"

79. Nos Galan @ Mountain Ash, Rhondda Valley.

NEVER before have I felt so nervous before a race. I was close to being physically sick as I paced up and down this narrow street in Mountain Ash on New Year's Eve. I was anxious before the London Marathon because of the pain which lay ahead, but I had trained hard, prepared properly and knew that I could do the job.

This was Nos Galan, a 5km race – not 26 miles. The difference was that this was a three-lap street race in front of thousands of spectators, and I was entered in the elite race. I was bricking it big time. The fear of being disgraced, a public humiliation as I trailed in dog last minutes behind the rest of the field of international runners, was at the forefront of my mind. "We've got a class field running this evening," announced the chirpy chappy over the Tannoy. "The leading runners should be through in around 14 minutes and the rest of the field in about 18 minutes." Geez! I have only once ever run under 20 minutes for a 5km race. With a lack of any speed training this past year I was hoping to finish somewhere between 21 and 22 minutes.

I looked at the other runners warming up in the street. They were all sporting the latest gear including super-fast, lightweight shoes. I was still running in one of the three pairs of Asics which had got me round the running year. There was no conversation, no passing smiles or nods of acknowledgement. These guys were in the zone – I was in the toilet!

But Nos Galan was a race I had to do. So much so, that I had constructed the most difficult of logistical exercises in order to run two races in five hours on the same day spread 170 miles apart on my final day of racing in 2007.

Nos Galan is a popular race through the streets of Mountain Ash in the Rhondda Valley which takes place every New Year's Eve. The race commemorates the legend that is Guto Nyth Bran, a man who could catch a bird in flight, chase and capture a hare in the field, and run from Porth to Pontypridd and back in the time it took to boil a kettle!

Guto, who was born in 1700, was the Linford Christie of his day, a man who worked on a farm, tending sheep, but who became famous in the vallies for his running prowess. He would regularly compete in races winning convincingly, and as the challengers became fewer and fewer, Guto chose to go into early retirement.

That was until a few years later when, at the age of 37, a new challenger persuaded Guto for a head-to-head race from Bedwas to Newport - a distance of 12 miles. Guto won the race in a remarkable time of 53 minutes (the current half marathon record is just under 59 minutes). However, in the celebrations which followed, Guto collapsed and died in the arms of his loved one, Sian-O'-Shop. He was carried to his final resting place at Llanwonno Church.

Guto's life is celebrated every year in Mountain Ash when a leading sportsman or woman visits Guto's grave to lay a wreath in recognition of his superhuman achievements before the start of the Nos Galan races. The identity of the celebrity is not revealed until just before the race. Among the mystery runners who have carried out the task are Ron Jones, David Hemery, Steve Jones, Kirsty Wade, Nicole Cooke, Neil Jenkins and Iwan Thomas, who was one of my guests at the Celebrity Question of Sport quiz. That sporting hero this year was Welsh rugby full-back Kevin Morgan who ran into the town square holding a lighted torch from the athlete's Llanwonno grave to light a beacon which signified the start of the races.

Mountain Ash is a small town lying on a hillside off the main road to Aberdare. It was sealed off for the evening for this carnival of running. There was a fun fair, street entertainers, children's races as well as the main adults' races; the elite race at seven o'clock, followed by the main 5km run half an hour later.

As the Stubbington Green snail stood on the start line, anyone looking at me could smell the fear. Liz was standing on the corner armed with a camera. Her words of reassurance had washed over me. This was going to be such a public humiliation on a three-lap course around tightly-packed streets. For the first time I ever I was going to come last.

A huge fireworks display delayed the start which only served to heighten the anxiety. Despite being stripped down to my racing gear on a dark December evening, it wasn't too cold, but the tension inside was burning. There was no friendly banter among the elite runners, no smiles exchanged. I was cruising for a bruising. Then when we did get going I was caught by the suddenness of the start, and it took me a good minute to settle.

Boy, was the pace fast. I knew I was going to have to run out of my skin to be competitive. I ran hard, I ran fast, trying to not be dispirited by the runners passing me like express trains.

Half way round the first of the three town centre laps we ran up this dark track by the railway line on a slight incline to a bollard where a marshal was standing and looped back. From here I could see whoever was behind me and was comforted by the sight of nine or ten runners adrift. There was no way they were going to pass me; my target was to draw in those in front. The crowd support was huge – one lady in a lilting Welsh voice shouted out "are you single?" as I ran past. She must have been drunk seeing the sight of this manic runner with spittle on his chin straining, every sinew in his body to run as fast as he could.

This was like a city centre race. We passed the finish funnel in the high street at the end of the first lap and continued on the tight and twisting course. I was trying my guts out, and that target of pushing on without allowing anyone to pass was the incentive I needed. The support was tremendous. I felt like a proper athlete, not that there was any disguising the fact that compared to the hares at the front I was a tortoise at the back. I held my form strongly and crossed the line in a time of 20 minutes 20 seconds. I was happy with the time, wishing it could have been 21 seconds faster, but delighted to have survived and not disgraced myself.

Liz walked over to congratulate me. I was so relieved and then the reality dawned that I had to get my arse into gear to get to Derbyshire. I still had one more race to go. We had parked the car out of town, so we were on our way down the A470 to Cardiff in pretty quick time – me driving, and Liz plying me with food and drink.

Fortunately, the roads were quiet on New Year's Eve. The M5 north only had light traffic, the speed cameras around Birmingham focussed minds for a brief while, and amazingly we arrived at our hotel in Derbyshire by 11pm. My dad was there to greet us with his friend Mary who had both travelled up to Milford by train that day.

There wasn't much time to exchange pleasantries since I needed to get changed and ready for the 80th and final race. Liz, Mary, my dad and myself, made the short walk from the hotel to the social club in the village which had been the starting point for this challenge a year earlier.

It felt strange to be here again 12 months on. Many times I had dreamt about this moment, the end of my epic adventure, but now the moment had arrived it possessed a dreamlike quality. A lot had happened in the past 12 months, I had experienced so much. Had it been worth it?

"People ask why I run. I say, If you have to ask, you will never understand. It is something only those select few know. Those who put themselves through pain, but know, deep down, how good it really feels"

EPILOGUE

SATURDAY, JANUARY 5th, 2008

IT IS a gloriously crisp Saturday morning, the fifth day of a new year when the view along the south coast is spectacular. This is home, this is my running manor, this is the tranquility of the Solent Way.

I look across towards the sleepy Isle of Wight as a huge container ship gently plies its way towards the port of Southampton, and the Red Jet catamaran skims across the water to Cowes. The air is a little nippy, every breath leaves a small vapour trail.

I'm picking a trail along the calf-sapping, knee-crunching shingle, 10 miles into a gentle training run with a group of friends. There's Richard Simms, who ran Race The Train in Wales with me the previous August, a time when we slogged our guts out on the Welsh hillsides and through the mud all in the vain hope of beating a steam train.

A few paces in front there is Marcus Lee, who has become a father since we battled our way on the eve of the London Marathon through the Worthing 20. With fatherhood, Marcus has become pretty adept at changing nappies like a Formula 1 racing team changes tyres. Leading the way up front, as ever, is Jon Leigh, a good mate who, like the rest of us, is a member of Stubbington Green Runners.

The only one missing of this regular Saturday morning training group is the Kimbernator, aka Nick Kimber, who has cried off with 'flu to miss out on the 15-mile training run. All three guys are building up for April's London Marathon. For me, this is my first run since New Year's Eve in Derbyshire.

Running another marathon couldn't be the furthest thought from my mind. In fact, reminded of Steve Redgrave's comments after winning gold at the Atlanta Olympics, shoot me if I run another marathon.

However on this gorgeous January day, I am simply loving it. I love running with friends again, catching up with gossip, sharing the latest corny jokes. I love running without pressure, because no matter how much I attempted to ignore the clock during the 80 race saga, trying not to worry about finishing as high up in the field as I could, once the starter's horn sounded those well-founded notions were ditched straight out of the window.

I love running along the Solent Way, a trail I have traced so many times. It has been my spiritual home, my confessional where I have cried over the tough times, agonised over making difficult decisions, and broken the stillness by screaming with joy when things have sometimes gone right.

Along the grass-topped cliffs, across the shingle of the beach, there is nothing quite as soothing as running by the sea.

There is a quiet spot along the shoreline along Southampton Water, overlooking Calshot Spit near the Hook with Warsash Nature Reserve, where one day I would like my ashes sprinkled. Then, legions of sweaty runners and walkers can stamp their size nines all over me!

Since finishing the challenge in Milford in the early hours of New Year's Day, it has all been a bit of an anti-climax. For days afterwards I felt exhausted and unwell. It was as if my body had been holding itself together for the past 12 months, resisting any injury or illness. But once I had crossed the finish line in Derbyshire at five minutes past midnight, so the floodgates of relief were breached. For days afterwards I didn't eat much, my body ached, I felt listless and lethargic.

I ran the Bryan Clifton Memorial Race a good minute faster than I had 12 months earlier.

From the start, half a dozen of the faster runners scorched down the road while I was content to settle in with a pleasantly brisk pace. Suddenly, I was passed by a child of no more than 10-years-old. He was running like kids do, free and with abandon, and with enormous reserves of stamina. "Come on dad," he cried, and suddenly dad flew past me, followed by his mum. What was this, a New Year's Eve family outing? The family turned out to be Shields family from Sheffield, with dad David and mum Jane, who incidentally represented Great Britain at the 10,000m in the 1988 Seoul Olympics.

I kept the Shields in my sights as we turned the half way mark at Duffield. By then, fireworks were exploding in the sky, a couple of cars drove past honking their horns soon followed by a fire engine heading towards Belper, blues and twos blaring.

"This is it, this really is it," I thought to myself on the home stretch. Frequently I have wondered how I would feel with the finish line in sight to my year-long adventure. At that moment in time I felt surprisingly detached and unemotional. No tears were welling similar to the choking emotions felt as I approached the end of the London Marathon, no fatigue or exhaustion suffered in the final miles of the Sleepwalker Midnight Marathon over the Brecon Beacons, none of the unmitigated joy at actually winning a race as I did when I cantered to victory at the immigration centre in Gosport.

This was clinical, this was job done. "Finish strongly and finish well," I told myself, as I eased past Jane up the final hill to finish just behind David for ninth place in 8 minutes 32 seconds to applause from the small crowd clustered outside the social club.

My dad was there to meet me along with Mary. I turned and jogged back down the road to join Liz and run in with her. She had been me with solidly throughout the year. I was thrilled she was there at the end to cross in 26th spot in a time of 11 minutes 18 seconds. "How do you fancy getting in the car and driving down to Cornwall to run the Brown Willy?" I joked, re-tracing our steps from exactly a year earlier. Her reply was unprintable.

The send-off at Milford was under-whelming. I wasn't expecting brass bands or bunting, but at least I thought there might have been some acknowledgement of the achievement. Instead, nothing was said.

Before the race I caught up with the race organiser, David Denton, who I had met 12 months earlier and we had spoken a few times since then. When I registered half an hour before the start to collect my race number, surprisingly he seemed totally disinterested.

"Where have you come from?" he asked coldly. "South Wales," I replied. There was no come-back or any questions about how they year had gone. I wasn't sure if David had registered who I was.

"You know I'm the fella who is running around the British Isles and this is my 80th and final race?"

"Yeah, I know," said David, scribbling something on his entry sheet. "I know someone who has run 60 odd races this year, and there is a guy who once ran more than 100!"

Oh thanks for the faint praise!

Liz had brought a bottle of champagne and party poppers with her, but it didn't feel right to celebrate. I just put my head in my hands glad it was all over. Moments later, I gathered up my clothes, and we walked out of the social club into the warm night air and back to our hotel.

Don't get me wrong, this whole challenge was not about ego, it was never about recognition, yet wherever I went in the British Isles race organisers and runners had been besides themselves with help and interest. They had gone to sometimes embarrassing lengths to publicise what I was doing, generous in their help towards my fund-raising.

Just days earlier, I had been given a whole page in the Derby Evening Telegraph publicising my adventure, giving fulsome praise and promotion to the Bryan Clifton Memorial Run. But from the race itself – nothing. If that sounds bitter, it's not meant to be. Possibly the feelings of disappointment.

The point, David, is that your friends may have run 60 or even 100 odd races in a year, but that is easy; one or two races a week. Anyone can do that if you want to run those events close to home. This challenge was unique. This was a challenge which no-one had done it before.

This was not a test of endurance, this was never an I-Spy book about how many races one person could tick off in a calendar year. If that was the case, I would have taken a year's sabbatical and tried to run 200 races in 12 months. Instead, this challenge was about running the length and breadth of the British Isles, competing in a huge variety of races of varying distances and terrain, meeting the characters and visiting some truly spectacular places.

It was about tracing the spirit of running, a culture which embraces and touches the lives of so many people and in so many different ways.

Meeting people like Mick Curry and his son Phil from Stratford-upon-Avon who he selflessly pushes round in a wheelchair, and Gay Eastoe from the Lake District who suffers from autism, but who still loves running and has raised more than £38,000 for charity, was humbling.

It has been about catching up with inspiring characters such as the legend that is athlete Ron Hill and round-the-world sailor, Dee Caffari.

But by and large, it has been about visiting ordinary folk the length and breadth of this nation, from Cape Wrath in the far north of Scotland, to Land's End, for whom running is a way of life.

What did I learn? I have met so many people, inspiring folk who don't sit in their comfort zone. Runners who, as Sir Chay Blyth once described to me, live life to the full and sail close to the edge. People for whom, when they look down at their gnarled feet the day they come to meet their maker, can truly say they achieved what they set out to do.

For me this was personal. I set out to do something which I was determined to finish it. It was about raising money for the Hampshire Autistic Society as well as raising awareness of autism wherever I went.

This was a voyage of discovery and without doubt the most worthwhile thing I have ever done.

"Pain is temporary, quitting is forever."

80 Races in One Year

The Races

1. Bryan Clifton Memorial Race

Where: Milford, Derbyshire.
When: December 31st.
Race time and placing: 9min 18sec / 11th (49 runners).
Distance: 2km.
2007 running mileage: 1.24 miles.
Round Britain travelling: 184 miles.
Race memento: Mug

2. Brown Willy 6

Where: Bodmin Moor, Cornwall.
When: January 1st.
Race time and placing: 1hr 6min 22sec / no placings – (250 runners).
Distance: 6.82 miles.
2007 running mileage: 8.06 miles.
Round Britain travelling: 642 miles.
Race memento: Framed picture of Brown Willy.

3. Tadworth 10

Where: Epsom Racecourse, Surrey.
When: January 7th.
Race time and placing: 1hr 15min 28sec / 112th (710).
Distance: 10 miles.
2007 running mileage: 18.06 miles.
Round Britain travelling: 783 miles.
Race memento: Pair of gloves.

4. Stubbington Green 10km.

Where: Stubbington Green, Hampshire.
When: January 14th.
Race time and placing: none.
Distance: 10km.
2007 running mileage: 18.06 miles.
Round Britain travelling: 793 miles.
Race memento: Mug.

5. Brass Monkey Half Marathon.

Where: York Racecourse, North Yorkshire.
When: January 21st.
Race time and placing: 1hr 34min 22sec / 275th (1010)
Distance: 13.1 miles.
2007 running mileage: 31.16 miles.
Round Britain travelling: 1,319 miles.
Race memento: Sweat shirt.

6. Not The Roman IX.

Where: Stratford-upon-Avon, Warwickshire.
When: January 28th.
Race time and placing: 52min 6sec / 92nd (588).
Distance: 7.43 miles.
2007 running mileage: 38.59 miles.
Round Britain travelling: 1,571 miles.
Race memento: Flint coaster.

7. Watford Half Marathon.

Where: Watford, Hertfordshire.
When: February 4th.
Race time and placing: 1hr 34min 55sec / 364th (1,947).
Distance: 13.1 miles.
2007 running mileage: 38.59 miles.
Round Britain travelling: 1,571 miles.
Race memento: T-shirt.

8. St Valentine's 30km.

Where: Stamford, Lincolnshire.
When: February 11th.
Race time and placing: 2hrs 21min 41sec / 156th (560).
Distance: 18.68 miles.
2007 running mileage: 57.27 miles.
Round Britain travelling: 1,905 miles.
Race memento: T-shirt.

9. St Peter's Great East Run.

Where: Bungay, Suffolk.
When: February 18th.
Race time and placing: 1hr 28min 51sec / 102nd (516).
Distance: 12.44 miles.
2007 running mileage: 69.71 miles.
Round Britain travelling: 2,313 miles.
Race memento: towel, drinks bottle, bottle of beer.

10. The Terminator.

Where: Pewsey, Wiltshire.
When: February 25th.
Race time and placing: 1hr 52min 42sec / 267th (740).
Distance: 11.49 miles.
2007 running mileage: 81.2 miles.
Round Britain travelling: 2,425 miles.
Race memento: T-shirt.

11. Vectis Lunatics Full Moon Hash.

Where: Ryde, Isle of Wight.
When: March 1st.
Race time and placing: 55 min 10sec / no placings.
Distance: 3.5 miles.
2007 running mileage: 84.7 miles.
Round Britain travelling: 2,466 miles.
Race memento: Post-race lemonade as part of a drinking contest.

12. Ballycotton 10.

Where: Ballycotton, County Cork, Republic of Ireland.
When: March 4th.
Race time and placing: 1hr 11min 56sec / 415th (1943).
Distance: 10 miles.
2007 running mileage: 94.7 miles.
Round Britain travelling: 3,166 miles.
Race memento: Mug.

13. Banbury 15.

Where: Banbury, Oxfordshire.
When: March 11th.
Race time and placing: 1hr 53min 41sec / 94th (380).
Distance: 15 miles.
2007 running mileage: 109.7 miles.
Round Britain travelling: 3,369 miles.
Race memento: Medal.

14. Glenariff Mountain Race.

Where: Glenariff, County Antrim, Northern Ireland.
When: March 17th.
Race time and placing: 1hr 6min 10sec / 51st (71).
Distance: 5.92 miles.
2007 running mileage: 115.62 miles.
Round Britain travelling: 3,750
Race memento: Sack of potatoes

15. Jimmy's 10

Where: Downpatrick, County Down, Northern Ireland.
When: March 18th.
Race time and placing: 43min 44sec / 90th (221)
Distance: 10km.
2007 running mileage: 121.82 miles.
Round Britain travelling: 4,142 miles.
Race memento: T-shirt, coaster, calculator.

16. Asics Coniston 14

Where: Coniston, Cumbria.
When: March 24th.
Race time and placing: 1hr 44min 37sec / 270th (1359)
Distance: 14 miles.
2007 running mileage: 135.82 miles.
Round Britain travelling: 4,772 miles.
Race memento: Coaster.

17. Worthing 20

Where: Worthing, West Sussex.
When: April 1st.
Race time and placing: 2hrs 33min 15sec / 128th (660).
Distance: 20 miles.
2007 running mileage: 155.82 miles.
Round Britain travelling: 4,862 miles.
Race memento: Towel.

18. Healthspan 10km

Where: Rovers AC, Port Soif, Guernsey.
When: April 6th.
Race time and placing: 44min 9sec / 87th (201)
Distance: 10km.
2007 running mileage: 162.02 miles.
Round Britain travelling: 4,988 miles.

19. Keith Falla Memorial Cross Country Race

Where: Les Amarreurs, Vale, Guernsey.
When: April 7th.
Race time and placing: 33min 48sec / 67th (128)
Distance: 4.75 miles.
2007 running mileage: 166.77 miles
Round Britain travelling: 4,996 miles

20. Guernsey Easter Running Festival 4x2 mile Cross Country Relay

Where: Les Amarreurs, Vale, Guernsey.
When: April 8th.
Race time and placing: 13min 45sec / 85th (152)
Distance: 2 miles.
2007 running mileage: 168.77 miles.
Round Britain travelling: 5,004 miles

21. Healthspan Half Marathon.

Where: St Peterport, Guernsey.
When: April 9th.
Race time and placing: 1hr 38min 27sec / 66th (144)
Distance: 13.1 miles.
Overall in Guernsey Easter Running Festival: 49th (76)
2007 running mileage: 181.87 miles.
Round Britain travelling: 5,222 miles.
Race memento (for four races): long-sleeved t-shirt.

22. Flitwick 10km

Where: Flitwick, Bedfordshire.
When: April 15th.
Race time and placing: 52min 00sec / 395th (788).
Distance: 10km.
2007 running mileage: 188.07 miles.
Round Britain travelling: 5,446 miles.
Race memento: medal.

23. Flora London Marathon.

Where: Blackheath to The Mall, London.
When: April 22nd.
Race time and placing: 3hrs 29min 24sec / 3,639th (35,674)
Distance: 26.2 miles.
2007 running mileage: 214.27 miles.
Round Britain travelling: 5,612 miles.
Race memento: medal & goody bag, including technical t-shirt.

24. Horton Bull Run.

Where: Horton, nr Chipping Sodbury, Gloucestershire.
When: April 29th.
Race time and placing: 29min 11sec / 27th (219)
Distance: 4 miles.
2007 running mileage: 218.27 miles.
Round Britain travelling: 5,818 miles.
Race memento: medal.

25. Dudley Kingswinford 10km.
Where: Dudley Kingswinford, West Midlands.
When: May 2nd.
Race time and placing: 45min 3sec / 241st (1099).
Distance: 10km.
2007 running mileage: 224.47 miles.
Round Britain travelling: 6,138 miles.
Memento: Glass goblet.

26. Round the Tree 3
Where: Torrington, Devon.
When: May 4th.
Race time and placing: 21min 57sec / 33rd (60).
Distance: 3 miles.
2007 running mileage: 227.67 miles.
Round Britain travelling: 6,466 miles.
Memento: a beer in the pub afterwards.

27. Neolithic Cani-X
Where: Stonehenge, Wiltshire.
When: May 6th.
Race time and placing: 32min 28sec / 7th (27).
Distance: 4 miles.
2007 running mileage: 231.67 miles.
Round Britain travelling: 6,570 miles.
Memento: medal and dog biscuits.

28. Penicuik 10km.
Where: Penicuik, Midlothian, Scotland.
When: May 12th.
Race time and placing: 44min 6sec / 70th (190).
Distance: 10km.
2007 running mileage: 237.87 miles.
Round Britain travelling: 6,939 miles.
Memento: medal.

29. Loch Eriboll Half Marathon.

Where: Durness, Lairg, Scotland.
When: May 14th.
Race time and placing: 1hr 38min 50sec / 19th (57).
Distance: 13.1 miles.
2007 running mileage: 250.97 miles.
Round Britain travelling: 7,204 miles.

30. Sangomore Hill Run.

Where: Durness, Lairg, Scotland.
When: May 15th.
Race time and placing: 41min 38sec / 24th (53)
Distance: 5.05 miles.
2007 running mileage: 256.02 miles
Round Britain travelling: 7,205 miles.

31. Round Durness Run.

Where: Durness, Lairg, Scotland.
When: May 16th.
Race time and placing: 1hr 5min 20sec / 17th (58).
Distance: 8.48 miles.
2007 running mileage: 264.5 miles.
Round Britain travelling: 7,208 miles.

32. Target Zero Run

Where: Durness, Lairg, Scotland.
When: May 17th.
Race time and placing: 24min 30sec / no placings.
Distance: 3 miles.
2007 running mileage: 267.5 miles.
Round Britain travelling: 7,211 miles.

33. Cape Wrath Marathon Relay.

Where: Durness, Lairg, Scotland.
When: May 19th.
Race time and placing: 1hr 18min 1sec / 2nd team.
Distance: 11.4 miles.
2007 running mileage: 278.9 miles.
Round Britain travelling: 7,831 miles.
Memento: T-shirt and goody bag.

34. Mull of Kintyre Half Marathon.
Where: Campbeltown, Argyll & Bute, Scotland.
When: May 27th.
Race time and placing: 1hr 35min 29sec / 21st (148).
Distance: 13.1 miles.
2007 running mileage: 292 miles.
Round Britain travelling: 8,815 miles.
Memento: medal.

35. Beat the Baton
Where: Battersea Park, London.
When: May 28th.
Race time and placing: 25min 30sec / no placings.
Distance: 5km.
2007 running mileage: 295.1 miles.
Round Britain travelling: 8,976 miles.
Memento: t-shirt.

36. South Downs Relay.
Where: Beachy Head, East Sussex to Chilcomb, near Winchester, Hampshire.
When: June 2nd.
Race time and placing: leg 3: 4.48 miles in 31min 37sec; leg 7: 5.52 miles in 40min 23sec; leg 13: 6.51 miles in 58min 27sec. Stubbington B team: 14hrs 15mins 10sec (7th of 9).
Distance: (race distance 100 miles) 16.51 miles.
2007 running mileage: 311.61 miles.
Round Britain travelling: 9,138 miles.
Memento: Memories of a bloomin' hard day.

37. Nike Blaydon Race.
Where: Newcastle to Blaydon, Tyneside.
When: June 9th.
Race time and placing: 41min 23sec / 515th (3,338).
Distance: 5.7 miles.
2007 running mileage: 317.31 miles.
Round Britain travelling: 9,478 miles.
Memento: t-shirt.

38. Potters Arf Marathon.

Where: Stoke-on-Trent, Staffordshire.
When: June 10th.
Race time and placing: 1hr 41min 8sec / 203rd (925).
Distance: 13.1 miles.
2007 running mileage: 330.41 miles.
Round Britain travelling: 9,864 miles.
Memento: t-shirt.

39. Freckleton Half Marathon.

Where: Freckleton, near Preston, Lancashire.
When: June 17th.
Race time and placing: 1hr 38min 2sec / 116th (497).
Distance: 13.1 miles.
2007 running mileage: 343.51 miles.
Round Britain travelling: 10,390 miles.
Memento: mug.

40. Humber Bridge Half Marathon.

Where: Hessle, East Riding, Yorkshire.
When: June 24th.
Race time and placing: 1hr 45min 43sec / 356th (1,137)
Distance: 13.1 miles.
2007 running mileage: 356.61 miles.
Round Britain travelling: 10,904 miles.
Memento: t-shirt and medal.

41. Summer Series Orienteering.

Where: Longmoor Training Camp, near Petersfield, Hampshire.
When: June 27th.
Race time and placing: 35min 2sec / 9th (45).
Distance: 4.5km.
2007 running mileage: 359.4 miles.
Round Britain travelling: 10,968 miles.
Memento: a well-handled orienteering map.

42. **Prestwold Hall 10km.**
Where: Prestwold Hall, near Loughborough, Leicestershire.
When: July 1st.
Race time and placing: 58min 18sec / 314th (375).
Distance: 10km.
2007 running mileage: 365.6 miles.
Round Britain travelling: 11,296 miles.
Memento: glass paperweight.

43. **Tickhill Gala run.**
Where: Tickhill, near Doncaster, South Yorkshire.
When: July 7th.
Race time and placing: 25min 14sec / 14th (44).
Distance: 3.5 miles.
2007 running mileage: 369.1 miles.
Round Britain travelling: 11,510 miles.
Memento: medal.

44. **Spilsby Show 6**
Where: Spilsby, near Louth, Lincolnshire.
When: July 8th.
Race time and placing: 48min 59sec / 74th (116)
Distance: 6 miles.
2007 running mileage: 375.1 miles.
Round Britain travelling: 11,788 miles.
Memento: glass paperweight.

45. **Wenlock Olympic Games**
Where: Much Wenlock, Shropshire.
When: July 15th.
Race time and placing: 51min 26sec / 40th (124).
Distance: 7 miles.
2007 running mileage: 382.1 miles.
Round Britain travelling: 12,132 miles.
Memento: medal.

46. Mug's Game 5

Where: Itchen Valley Country Park, Eastleigh, Hampshire.
When: July 21st.
Race time and placing: none.
Distance: 4.5 miles.
2007 running mileage: 382.1 miles.
Round Britain travelling: 12,144 miles.
Memento: mug.

47. Swanage Half Marathon:

Where: Swanage, Dorset.
When: July 28th.
Race time and placing: 1hr 46min 15sec / 90th (280).
Distance: 13.1 miles.
2007 running mileage: 395.2 miles.
Round Britain travelling: 12,273 miles.
Memento: medal.

48. Harlow 10

Where: Harlow, Essex.
When: August 5th.
Race time and placing: 1hr 19min 27sec / 138th (296).
Distance: 10 miles.
2007 running mileage: 405.2 miles.
Round Britain travelling: 12,517 miles.
Memento: t-shirt.

49. Mynyddislwyn Mile

Where: Mynyddislwyn, Newbridge, Gwent.
When: August 10th.
Race time and placing: 12min 15sec / 32nd (47).
Distance: One mile.
2007 running mileage: 406.2 miles.
Round Britain travelling: 12,768 miles.
Memento: Post-race bottle of cider or beer.

50. Isle of Man Half Marathon.
Where: Ramsey, Isle of Man.
When : August 12th.
Race time and placing: 1hr 38min 15sec / 40th (213).
Distance: 13.1 miles.
2007 running mileage: 419.3 miles.
Round Britain travelling: 13,230 miles.
Memento: t-shirt, medal and goody bag (with Mars bar!).

51. St Levan 10km.
Where: St Levan, near Penzance, Cornwall.
When: August 17th.
Race time and placing: 46min 33sec / 71st (181).
Distance: 10km.
2007 running mileage: 425.5 miles.
Round Britain travelling: 13,471 miles.
Memento: medal.

52. Race the Train.
Where: Tywyn, Gwynedd, Mid Wales.
When: August 18th.
Race time: 2hrs 9mins 20sec / 306th (689).
Distance: 14.75 miles.
2007 running mileage: 440.25 miles.
Round Britain travelling: 14,068 miles.
Memento: t-shirt, medal and goody bag (included Beef jerky and tea bags).

53. Battle of Sedgemoor 10km
Where: Langport, Somerset.
When: August 26th.
Race time: 50min 51sec / 202nd (377).
Distance: 10km.
2007 running mileage: 446.45 miles.
Round Britain travelling: 14,269 miles.
Memento: towel.

54. Braemar Highland Games – Morrone Hill Race.
Where: Braemar, Royal Deeside, Scotland.
When: September 1st.
Race time: 41min 16sec / 55th (71).
Distance: 3.3 miles.
2007 running mileage: 449.75 miles.
Round Britain travelling: 14,794 miles.
Memento: nothing.

55. freshnlo Great Scottish Run
Where: Glasgow, Scotland.
When: September 2nd.
Race time: 1hr 39min 18sec / 946th (6446).
Distance: 13.1 miles.
2007 running mileage: 462.85 miles.
Round Britain travelling: 15,252 miles.
Memento: Medal, t-shirt and goody bag.

56. Test Way Relay
Where: Stockbridge, Hampshire.
When: September 3rd.
Race time: 42min 41sec (relay – 13th out of 13 teams).
Distance: 5.74 miles.
2007 running mileage: 468.59 miles.
Round Britain travelling: 15,319 miles.
Memento: nothing.

57. The Grizzly
Where: Seaton, Devon.
When: September 4th.
Race time: 3hrs 44min 55sec / 428th (996 runners).
Distance: 19.7 miles.
2007 running mileage: 488.29 miles.
Round Britain travelling: 15,517 miles.
Memento: t-shirt.

58. Round Norfolk Relay.
Where: King's Lynn, Norfolk.
When: September 15th.
Race time: 2hrs 9min 40sec (relay – 47th out of 50 teams).
Distance: 16.63 miles.
2007 running mileage: 504.92 miles.
Round Britain travelling: 15,886 miles.
Memento: t-shirt and glass paperweight.

59. Sleepwalker Midnight Marathon.
Where: Talybont on Usk, Brecon, South Wales.
When: September 22nd.
Race time: 3hrs 54mins 16sec / 11th (50).
Distance: 20 miles.
2007 running mileage: 524.92 miles.
Round Britain travelling: 16,214 miles.
Memento: certificate.

60. Ron Hill Birthday 5km Race.
Where: Littleborough, near Rochdale, Lancashire.
When: September 27th.
Race time: 22min 38sec / 100th (173)
Distance: 5km
2007 running mileage: 528.02 miles.
Round Britain travelling: 16,724 miles.
Memento: nothing.

61. BUPA Great North Run.
Where: Newcastle-upon-Tyne, Tyne & Wear.
When: September 30th.
Race time: 1hr 37min 00sec / 1,722nd (50,000).
Distance: 13.1 miles.
2007 running mileage: 541.12 miles.
Round Britain travelling: 17,396 miles.
Memento: medal, t-shirt and goody bag.

62. Chiquita Bananaman Run.
Where: Willen Lake, Milton Keynes, Buckinghamshire.
When: October 7th.
Race time: 47min 37sec / 19th (400).
Distance: 10km.
2007 running mileage: 547.32 miles.
Round Britain travelling: 17,642 miles.
Memento: t-shirt and medal.

63. IRC Haslar 10km Run.
Where: Haslar Immigration Removal Centre, Gosport, Hampshire.
When: October 11th.
Race time: 46min 28sec / 1st (13).
Distance: 10km.
2007 running mileage: 553.52 miles.
Round Britain travelling: 17,664 miles.
Memento: medal.

64. Swindon Half Marathon.
Where: Swindon, Wiltshire.
When: October 14th.
Race time: 1hr 37min 6sec / 140th (1,058).
Distance: 13.1 miles
2007 running mileage: 566.62 miles.
Round Britain travelling: 17,816 miles.
Memento: medal.

65. Bushy Park Time Trial.
Where: Bushy Park, Hampton Court, Middlesex.
When: October 20th.
Race time: 20min 54sec / 69th (336).
Distance: 3.1 miles
2007 running mileage: 569.72 miles.
Round Britain travelling: 17,963 miles.
Memento: t-shirt.

66. Stroud Half Marathon.

Where: Stroud, Gloucestershire.
When: October 21st:
Race time: 1hr 37min 4sec / 403 (1,161).
Distance: 13.1 miles.
2007 running mileage: 582.82 miles.
Round Britain travelling: 18,166 miles.
Memento: medal

67. BUPA Great South Run.

Where: Portsmouth, Hampshire.
When: October 28th.
Race time: 1hr 34min 19sec / 5,602 (12,000).
Distance: 10 miles.
2007 running mileage: 592.82 miles.
Round Britain travelling: 18,195 miles.
Memento: medal, t-shirt and goody bag.

68. Guy Fawkes 10.

Where: Ripley Castle, Harrogate, Yorkshire.
When: November 4th.
Race time: 1hr 18min 49sec / 262nd (828).
Distance: 10 miles.
2007 running mileage: 602.82 miles.
Round Britain travelling: 18,761 miles.
Memento: t-shirt and goody bag with chocolate and tea!

69. Grand Union Canal Half Marathon.

Where: Cowley, Middlesex to Watford, Hertfordshire.
When: November 11th.
Race time: 1hr 38min 13sec / 46th (285).
Distance: 13.1 miles.
2007 running mileage: 615.92 miles.
Round Britain travelling: 18,936 miles.
Memento: medal.

70. Brampton to Carlisle Race.
Where: Brampton to Carlisle, Cumbria.
When: November 17th .
Race time: 1hr 10min 40sec / 270th (613)
Distance: 10 miles.
2007 running mileage: 625.92 miles.
Round Britain travelling: 19,398 miles.
Memento: nothing.

71. Gill Pimblott Memorial 5km Race.
Where: Gin Pit Village, Tyldesley, Greater Manchester.
When: November 18th.
Race time: 23min 3scc / 41st (102)
Distance: 5km
2007 running mileage: 629.02 miles.
Round Britain travelling: 19,628 miles.
Memento: medal.

72. Leeds Abbey Dash.
Where: Leeds City Centre, Yorkshire.
When: November 25th.
Race time: 42min 34sec / 648th (6,000)
Distance: 10km
2007 running mileage: 635.22 miles.
Round Britain travelling: 20,154 miles.
Memento: t-shirt.

73. Liverpool Santa Dash.
Where: Liverpool city centre, Merseyside.
When: December 2nd.
Race time: 27min 30sec (placing unknown among 6,000 Santas!)
Distance: 5km
2007 running mileage: 638.32 miles.
Round Britain travelling: 20,642 miles.
Memento: t-shirt and medal.

74. **Keyworth Turkey Trot.**
Where: Keyworth, Nottinghamshire.
When: December 9th.
Race time: 1hr 38min 6sec / 195th (762)
Distance: 13.1 miles
2007 running mileage: 651.42 miles.
Round Britain travelling: 21,027 miles.
Memento: Mini thermos flask.

75. **Merthyr Mawr Christmas Pud.**
Where: Merthyr Mawr, Bridgend, Glamorgan.
When: December 16th.
Race time: 51min 36sec / 219th (630)
Distance: 5.7 miles.
2007 running mileage: 657.12 miles.
Round Britain travelling: 21,349 miles.
Memento: Christmas pudding, coaster and food goodies.

76. **Christmas Pudding Dash.**
Where: Battle, East Sussex.
When: December 22nd.
Race time: 36min 48sec / 36th (220)
Distance: 5 miles.
2007 running mileage: 662.12 miles.
Round Britain travelling: 21,529 miles.
Memento: Christmas pudding.

77. **Round the Lakes 10k.**
Where: Poole, Dorset.
When: December 26th
Race time: 52min 26sec / 241st (335)
Distance: 10km.
2007 running mileage: 668.32 miles.
Round Britain travelling: 21,622 miles.
Memento: Bottle of wine.

78. Maldon Mud Race.

Where: Maldon, Essex.
When: December 30th
Race time: 10min 17sec / 69th (181)
Distance: @ 400 metres.
2007 running mileage: 668.32 miles.
Round Britain travelling: 21,911 miles.
Memento: Nothing.

79. Nos Galan

Where: Mountain Ash, Rhondda Valley, South Wales.
When: December 31st
Race time: 20min 27sec / 39th (49).
Distance: 5km
2007 running mileage: 671.42 miles.
Round Britain travelling: 22,070 miles.
Memento: t-shirt and medal.

80. Bryan Clifton Memorial Race.

Where: Milford, Derbyshire.
When: December 31st
Race time: 8min 32sec / 9th (31).
Distance: 2km
2007 running mileage: 672.66 miles.
Round Britain travelling: 22,448 miles.
Memento: nothing.

Honours Board

Favourite race: Coniston 14.

Worst race: Grand Union Half.

Hardest race: Sleepwalker Midnight Marathon.

Most scenic: Cape Wrath Challenge.

Ugliest race: Prestwood 10k & Stroud Half Marathon.

Best atmosphere: Great North Run.

Worst atmosphere: freshnlo Great Scottish Run

Best value: Guy Fawkes 10 & Merthyr Mawr Christmas Pud.

Worst value: Brampton to Carlisle 10.

Most over-rated: Brass Monkey Half Marathon.

Most under-rated: Bushy Park Time Trial.

Best organised: Freckleton Half Marathon & Swindon Half Marathon.

Worst organised: Humber Bridge Half Marathon.

Most satisfying: Flora London Marathon.

Best memento: Towel at Battle of Sedgemoor 10km

Most unusual memento: Sack of potatoes from the Glenariff Mountain Race.

Best mug: Race The Train.

Running, to me, is more than just a physical exercise...it's a consistent reward for victory!

And Finally...

PROMISES....this will not be a Gwyneth Paltrow moment from the Oscars, with gushing tears and an endless list of people to thank, but now I have reached the end of this journey it is important to highlight those who have been there along the way.

In any case, if you're not featured, you're not going to read this anyway!

I want to say thanks to:

Liz Hall: my partner and companion throughout the year, who took part in 26 of the 80 races. Absolutely brilliant. She hated my driving, but was always there for me with advice, encouragement and a pack of fruit pastilles!

Micah, Leo and Ross: who had to put up with an absent dad for most of 2007 but gave me excellent support.

Thanks to Rae for your patience.

Sally Hillycar: we first threw around this idea in 2006 and amazingly it all came together. A good friend and wonderful support. It wouldn't have happened without you. Profiteroles!

Gemma Harvey and Kerry James: along with Sally, the glamour girls from the fund-raising department at the Hampshire Autistic Society who organised several events during the year and were patient throughout, despite all my hassling.

Gary Littlecott: great mate and training partner, who kept me going whatever the weather.

Andy Puntis: artist extraordinaire with the Southern Daily Echo in Southampton who helped put together the graphics and picture pages in this book.

Editor Ian Murray and the Southern Daily Echo team: thanks for all your support and encouragement too during the year. Did I ever turn up for work?!

Mum and dad: their support during moments of major doubt and extreme trepidation was key. As for the Kendal Mint Cake at the 20-mile mark of the London Marathon, dad, that was a life-saver! Thanks for all the proof-reading too.

Flybe: flew me and my bags round the British Isles and made a huge difference to the travelling.

Haywood Office Solutions, HudsonCooper, Asics, Fone Trader: fantastic sponsors and very enthusiastic supporters.

Brian Richardson: with the help of his team at HMS Temeraire, the ex-Gladiator contestant put together a superb sports day, despite the rain.

Will Feebery: an inspirational man, one of the best, who was always there to help. A fantastic master of ceremonies for the sportsman's dinner.

Mike Bell: first class photographer and fantastic help with a lot of the promotional literature.

Nick & Helen Kimber, Malcolm Price, Eryl Penney, Paul & Marj Hammond, Di & James Hammersley: thanks for your help in organising the Mug's Game 5 race.

Alan Marsh (Pompey Joggers), Pete Staunton (Just Run), Richard Dean, St John Ambulance, Rachel Odell (Itchen Valley Country Park): helped put on a great day at Itchen Valley.

Matt Le Tissier, Jason Dodd, Dee Caffari, Iwan Thomas, Shaun Udal, John Crawley, Chris Wilkinson, George Burley, Conor O'Shea, Gordon Watson: celebrity support all the way throughout the year, thanks a lot guys.

Peter Hood: a top man who hosted the celebrity Question of Sport and Any Sporting Questions fund-raiser at the Rose Bowl.

Simon Tooley: the south coast's top quizmaster who made the Question of Sport evening such a success.

Steve Power: Wave 105 breakfast time DJ, a great supporter who, with a smile, masterminded his way through a very wet sports day where he was master of ceremonies,

Jon Cuthill: BBC Radio Solent presenter who kept the fund-raising and the publicity rolling throughout 2007.

Kuti Miah: hosted a wonderful curry night at his Southampton restaurant as a finale to the fund-raising year.

Afrodisiac: the fantastic all-girl singing group of Sammi, Charmaine and Laura, who reached the X-Factor Boot Camp, and should have gone on further. They were awesome with their performance at Kuti's.

Trophyman: the Southampton-based company were very generous in support with medals and trophies for some of the fund-raising challenges.

Nova International: thanks to David Hart and Nicola Hedley for arranging entries to the Great Run series of races.

John Walshe (Ballycotton 10), Brian Porter (Freckleton Half), Joe Quinn (Downpatrick 10km), Bob Houston (Blaydon Races): four race directors who were especially helpful, but thank you to all the race organisers for their time and generosity at each of the events.

Doug and Sally Reid: wonderful company and accommodation in the heart of the glorious Leicestershire countryside.

Ron Hill: the great man kindly gave up his afternoon to chat about his legendary running career, and made a darn good cup of tea too.

Mark Alexander and family: thanks for putting up with me during my St Patrick's weekend in Northern Ireland.

Andy and Diane Hammersley: Liz's brother and sister-in-law who kindly looked after us for a couple of trips to Yorkshire.

Angela Anderson: The owner of Elyseum Health & Beauty in Whiteley near Southampton, who had the dubious pleasure of waxing my legs for charity.

Jenny Davies: gave me a valuable insight into diet and nutrition for the year.

Mark Diment: a superb physio who got me through a year of running injury-free.

Rick Pearson (P-Rick) and Deanna (Bumps): Isle of Wight hashers, great company, who allowed me to borrow their dog Boykie for the Neolithic Cani-X.

Stubbington Green Runners and Southampton Running Club: thanks to all my friends at both clubs for their support during the year, especially those who ran with me at races.

Garry Perratt: the excellent organiser of Axe Valley Runners' fearsome Grizzly, whose inspiring quotes of note signs are dotted around the picturesque Devon course. This provided the idea for the quotes which are sprinkled about this book. Garry rifled through his garage to jot down the thought-provoking and numerous messages for me. These and many other quotes are drawn from a huge variety of sources too numerous to mention.

Thank you to the many photographers who have allowed me to use their photographs copyright free in this book. Theirs was an extremely generous gesture, to which I am very grateful for.

So it is sincere thanks to:

Derek Haden Photography (Suffolk): www.derekhaden.com

Graham Russell Photography (Surrey): www.grahamrussell.info

Southern Daily Echo (Southampton): www.dailyecho.co.uk

Mike Bell Photography (Southampton): www.mikebell.co.uk

Alan Worth Photographic (Leicester): www.a-w-p.com

See Me In Action Sports Photography (Salisbury): www.seemeinaction.co.uk

SportCam (Surrey): www.sportcam.net

Stephen Armstrong (Ballymena, Northern Ireland): Stephen@carn86.freeserve.co.uk

Mark McGloughlin (Ballycotton, Republic of Ireland): www.picturethis.ie
Down Democrat (Downpatrick, Northern Ireland): www.downdemocrat.com
Mick Hall Photography (Staffordshire): www.mickhall-photos.com
AntBliss.com Digital Photos (Sussex): www.AntBliss.com
Marathonfoto: www.marathonfoto.com
Swindon Advertiser: www.swindonadvertiser.co.uk
Maldon & Burnham Standard: www.maldonandburnhamstandard.co.uk
Brackla Harriers (Bridgend, Wales): www.brackla-harriers.org
Isle of Man Photos (Bill Dale): www.isleofmanphotos.com/
Banbury Guardian: www.banburyguardian.co.uk
Kevin Arrowsmith (Cape Wrath, Scotland): www.kevinarrowsmith.com
James Pyne Photography (Devon): www.jamespyne.co.uk
Courtwood Photographic (Land's End): www.courtwood.co.uk
Leukaemia Research: www.bananaman10k.com

....and thank you to everyone who supported and sponsored me during the year. Every bit of support was cherished and proved valuable in making 2007 a running success.

About the Author

Dave King has been a journalist for more years than he cares to remember and is currently editor of the Swindon Advertiser. This is his first foray into the wacky world of book-writing...and probably his last!

Dave lives in Hampshire and Wiltshire, and has three boys – Micah, Leo and Ross. Besides his twin passions of running and autism, he also has an unhealthy interest in following the plummeting fortunes of Notts County Football Club, reading trashy novels and listening to music best suited to the tone deaf.

Printed in the United States
209557BV00002B/6/P

9 781434 365552